Keep Your Joints Young

Banish your aches, pains and creaky joints

Sarah Key

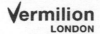

Vermilion
LONDON

3 5 7 9 10 8 6 4 2

Published in 2009 by Vermilion, an imprint of Ebury Publishing
Previously published in Australia as *Body In Action* by Allen & Unwin in 2006

Ebury Publishing is a Random House Group company

The Random House Group Limited Reg. No. 954009

Addresses for companies within the Random House Group can be found at
www.rbooks.co.uk

A CIP catalogue record for this book is available from the British Library

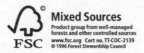

Mixed Sources
Product group from well-managed
forests and other controlled sources
www.fsc.org   Cert no. TT-COC-2139
© 1996 Forest Stewardship Council
FSC

The Random House Group Limited supports The Forest Stewardship Council
(FSC), the leading international forest certification organisation. All our titles that
are printed on Greenpeace approved FSC certified paper carry the FSC logo. Our
paper procurement policy can be found at

Printed in the UK by CPI Mackays, Chatham, ME5 8TD

ISBN 9780091929480

Copies are available at special rates for bulk orders. Contact the
sales development team on 020 7840 8487 for more information.

To buy books by your favourite authors and register for offers, visit
www.rbooks.co.uk

Contents

Figures acknowledgments

Figure on p. 20 is reprinted from *The Biomechanics of Back Pain*, Adams, Bogduk, Burton and Dolan, p. 17, © 2002, with permission from Elsevier.

Figure on p. 35 is reprinted from *Common Vertebral Joint Problems*, Grieve, p. 271, © 1985, with permission from Elsevier.

Figures on p. 61, p. 86, p. 91 and p. 100 are reprinted from *The Physiology of the Joints*, Kapandji, p. 141, p. 193, p. 209 and p. 251 respectively, © 1974, with permission from Elsevier.

Figures by Philip Wilson: on pp. 19, 22, 24, 25, 30, 36 and 43.

Figures by Ian Faulkner: on pp. 72 and 97.

Introduction

THE PERFECT STATE

The other day I was driving at dawn along one of Sydney's forest-fringed outer highways. It was one of those leafy dappled mornings of high summer with the occasional shaft of sunlight bursting through the greenery and making explosions of light wherever it landed. In the middle, cleaving its way through the foliage, ran my highway; a dusky blue thread of bitumen blending and becoming as one with the waking forest. As I rounded a corner I came upon a cyclist meandering at ease across the nearside lane of the roadway. I hung back to look because his actions had a compelling quality of beauty to them; a languid mark of excellence that made me want to stay and watch rather than speed on past. I kept my distance, watching transfixed as he acted out in front of me a perfect virtuoso performance of coordinated movement.

He was one of those men at the peak of physical fitness with the casual, confident swagger of one who is very sure of his own body's ability, and he was taking a breather. He dawdled and dreamed, back-pedalled and freewheeled, while he soaked in some of the breathy calm of the early day. He held the handlebars loosely with his left hand, and in one deft movement, reached down and unsnapped the water bottle from the diagonal bar of the bike frame. And then with the same casual ease, the gentle finesse of a ballerina and the accuracy of a marksman, he raised the water bottle high over his head, tilted his face back and squeezed a steady stream of water down into his open

1

mouth. All the time his legs pumping slowly, effortlessly pushing the pedals around.

I motored on past and soon enough came out into the harsh silver glare of the morning sun, where there were no cool chasms of green to give shade to the memory. But even now, long after, my mind is etched with the indelible picture of the man in the forest, the calm, the control, the timing, the elegant relaxed abandon every bit as seductive as the gymnast on the balance beam or the soccer player before the goal. Yet this man was lost in his own private reverie, oblivious to the incidental beauty of the way he was doing things. He had no idea of the unwitting quality of his performance, so breathlessly watched by this unknown admirer. He had no idea that his actions were the quintessence of human motor skills. He was out in the forest to watch the day breaking and to get his blood racing. To him, his superior coordination skills were a simple by-product of his search for fitness. And yet, he had it all—the human body at its best—long before age starts to nibble at the corners of prowess.

We can all catch glimpses of excellence like this if we take the time to look, snatches of it where we least expect to see. Everyday minutiae, there to be celebrated; beauty in motion it is called. You can see it by standing back and looking at anyone at the peak of their ability. They don't have to be the more obvious deliverers of excellence: the ballet dancer with her deliberately choreographed *pas de deux*, or the Olympic speed skater with his prowling feline grace. There is beauty in motion with a butcher wielding his knife. Free-flowing and precise, he stands back like a conductor of a symphony orchestra and cuts swathes of ham off the bone. Or the twirl and swirl of a window cleaner who cleans a plate-glass window with a single swipe—at its best perhaps one of the finest examples of beauty in economy of motion you will ever see.

The human body is a sublime piece of machinery that towers over its narrow base doing all manner of activities and hardly ever toppling over. If we take the time to look, we can see our own human frames acting out performances of fluent muscle effort, sliding and gliding through space in a symphony motion. Yet we rarely have any knowledge of the machinery that underlies this beautifully unselfconscious movement, of the interplay of dynamic systems that make our everyday movements so effortless. They just seem to happen as part of everyday life, with all of us assuming they will go on forever.

THE IMPERFECT STATE

The human skeleton is a supremely competent structure. It is upright, strong and agile and enables us to do an extraordinary variety of things. What keeps us and functioning usefully is our superior neuro-muscular control. This means that at one level our brain tells us what to do but at a lower level it instructs our postural muscles simply to keep us vertical so that we can do all those other useful things. I say 'simply' but really it isn't simple at all; it is a feat of insuperable grandeur. It is only that, when compared with other complex acts such as playing a cello (let alone reading the score), it is a simple act to stay upright.

But we do get it wrong, and our skeleton can develop problems. We encumber our postural mechanism with a heavy yoke of lassitude and bad habits, so we develop a list, even as we stand there. We lose our dynamic uprightness and start to bend and bow in all the wrong places.

Think of the skeleton as a ship's mast. As we stand tall, we are kept perpendicular by a collection of forward, aft and lateral stays to keep the mast balanced. The stays in this instance are the muscles, which work the levers (bones) and keep them straight. But the human frame is slightly more complicated than a ship's mast. For a start, the spine is divided into segments, with each of those segments able to move independently. So, it is a hard job to keep the human mast correctly aligned, especially when habits of poor posture and move-ment cause the muscular stays to become unequal in length and strength. Our mast develops a bow.

This comes about for several reasons. The foremost is that we do everything bent. Our 'doing actions' of precision function take place in a hunched-over posture so we can focus on the task at hand. The result over time is that we develop a subtle lean and our skeleton loses its dynamic balance. It may not be all that obvious—you may not *look* bowed as you stand there (although some people do)—it's just that you may find you can touch your toes easily enough but when it comes to bending back the other way, you can barely get beyond vertical. This is the first flaw—a critical flaw—and it is this inflexibility that sets the stage for difficulties in our lesser joints later on: the jaw, the knee, the shoulder or even the big toe.

If mother skeleton fails to stand upright, then all her joints become hampered in their daily toil. If the joints are off balance they don't run as well. A simple parallel, though perhaps a fanciful one, is of a skyscraper standing at an angle in the sky. All the internal machinery will work at a disadvantage. The elevators won't run smoothly up and down their shafts, the doors and windows won't open properly, the desks will inch across the floors. Just as well the leaning tower at Pisa doesn't have elevators. The truism is, the better your joints run, the better you run.

The next factor that encourages our curled-over stance is the general dearth of variety in the way we do things. Not only do we tend to do all our activities bent over, we don't do anything much else. We do the same things, in the same ways, at the same times, every day, forever and a day. Creatures of habit, we even get up at the same time every morning. We make the same movement to get out of bed (perhaps the most taxing activity of the day): we bend over the hand basin to turn the tap on, put our foot on the stool to tie the shoelaces, and we push buttons to make things happen. Invariably the whole day runs as a series of unvarying physical habits. Our workbenches are set at the right height and we don't even put our hand out of the car window any more to make a signal—the indicator lever is only a centimetre or two from the steering wheel. Variety is the exception rather than the rule and this meagreness of variety leads to trouble.

We could compensate for the usual flexed postures of precision work if we did more antidote actions to balance the time spent crumpled. But we don't.

At the end of the day we sit hunched in a sofa. We may get up to mooch across the room but it is reluctant and lacks romp—no verve, no spring, no Nijinski leaps. Even after a taxing period spent reading the paper, we rarely arch backwards; we rarely extend our spines and take our arms up behind our head and s-t-r-e-t-c-h back and away. We remain locked in by our stereotyped patterns and our joints become trapped by our physical habits.

This lack of flourish in our movements means that joint function is steadily reduced to its slimmest repertoire. The same old actions time and again—the hand to mouth but rarely behind the back; legs back and forth to walk but rarely knees to chin, and never the splits! Like the old wives' tale of our wide-eyed childhood, the wind changing to make permanent the grimace—only this time it's our joints getting fixed, not our face. Our joints crimp and lose freedom to go where they hardly ever go. The soft tissues quietly shrink and lose the capacity to get there, even if you want them to. Joint action loses opportunity, loses variety, loses lubrication, loses elastic stretch and even loses its clothing of muscle tissue. When joint action dries up, pain is but a whisker away.

For each part of the body a specific variety of actions predominate. Our joints develop a penchant for doing only their main thing and letting their lesser actions lapse. Whether you are a rice grower in China or an Inuit from Greenland, you tend to use your body in the same way, arms doing arm things and backs doing back things. Our Western lifestyle makes skeletal immobility worse because mod cons have wiped out much of the variety in the way we do things (before we had vacuum cleaners we had to heave the rug over the clothesline and bash it with a stick, or wring the clothes by hand!).

Universal patterns of movement make our skeletons all kink similarly and each joint has its own predestined sequence it follows when it comes to losing play. A hip kinks in its own hip way, failing to extend backwards or sideways, away from the other leg; a knee to swivel and fully straighten. As different as we all are in our body build, our habits, our weight, our fitness, our jobs or leisure, each particular joint deteriorates in all of us in the same way. And it doesn't matter whether you are a high jumper, a farmer or an office worker, every joint, when it starts to go, will follow its pattern and lose the same actions first.

The root cause of cumulative joint problems is the lack of variety in the way we use our bodies. That's the nuts and bolts of it. But what adds insult to this chronic state of unpreparedness is another set of factors: repetition or overuse of the movements we *do* make. We either do too little or too much; that is, we alternate between indolence and overactivity—a bad combination. Sport is usually the offender here but so too is the occasional bout of activity in the desert of non-activity; suddenly leaping up from the sofa to do a spate of shoveling in the garden. The skeleton struggles to accommodate the quantum leap from non-activity to repetitive aggressive over-activity. Maybe because the skeleton *seems* to cope so uncomplainingly we assume it will go on doing so indefinitely.

A smooth-running joint can be thrown by being victim to one dominant muscle group. It will be wrenched and yanked in a subtle repetitive way. This happens particularly in sports, such as tennis or golf, which consist of regimentally defined patterns of movement. The serve in tennis demands absolute adherence to the same pattern, over and over again. Your aim is to ace your opponent by making as precise a movement as possible. While there is the backhand and a limited range of forehand strokes to add variety, this is not the case with golf. Golf requires the same swing, in the same direction, with as much clout as you can muster. You can imagine what that does to your skeleton: nothing immediately disastrous and nothing that cannot be undone, but it sets up a whispering discord in your joints, which your skeleton then has to struggle to smooth over.

It is bad enough to have a skeleton that bows as you stand there, shoulders hunched forward and belly poking out, but it is even worse to have that skeleton beset by a patchy scatter of muscle groups, some too strong and others too loose. The bowing of the skeleton will be made worse if, going back to the analogy of the ship's mast, the front stays are too weak and the back ones too tight. Think of a puppet. It has a hard job functioning well if some strings pull easily while others don't, if some strings are too short while others too long. The result is a clonking subtle discord. What is true of the puppet is also true of our skeleton.

Balanced, properly coordinated muscular control is the very essence of healthy movement. Our joints are human hinges that permit movement between one bone and the next. In the perfect state, they form a perfectly poised dynamic system. They bend and straighten with effortless ease, the speed of movement and degree of bend controlled by the muscles. Every muscle performing a set movement has a partner to perform the reverse movement. For easy action, both need to be well-matched in length and strength. Take the knee, for example. The hamstrings bend the knee, the quadriceps at the front of the thigh straighten it. If both groups are equally balanced the knee can be nursed through the most extravagant explosions of movement. If they are not well-paired the knee can suffer easily, even with the most paltry of exertions. If the hamstrings are tight and do not allow the knee to straighten fully and, at the same time, the thigh muscles are weak and unable to match the hamstrings in their obstinacy, it is easy to tweak the knee. You may find you go down on the sports field without being tackled, or in the supermarket turning to fetch the marmalade.

When we are young, or even in later life if we are particularly lithe and skeletally well-balanced, the body does not hurt itself so easily. That's when our skeleton is covered with well-paired muscle groups and all the joints display a fine elastic quality: the springiness that young gymnasts demonstrate to a superlative degree. Muscles and joints can perform at their best: they can act powerfully and absorb shock without incident. But as we get older, repetitive and stereotyped movements upset this balance. A joint will be pinched by being in the grip of one dominant muscle in the pair. This takes time to manifest but sooner or later the joint will start running out of kilter. Insidious chafing and knocking will start. In a nutshell, incompetent muscle balance exposes a joint to greater wear and tear.

You might not realise this in the early stages. You may be unaware that a joint is starting to run hot from the subtle grind of not running true. You may only realise somewhere down the track when debility or even pain creeps in. Then it will dawn on you that the odd movement is uncomfortable—there's a pain in your forearm when shaking hands, difficulty getting your arm into your coat, or a tightness in one knee when you squat on your haunches. It is possible that you might recognise that something is wrong before the pain starts if you have your wits about you. You might notice that one arm is failing to go up as high as the other above your head, or that your knees are starting to click and grate whenever you bend. But these changes are mostly creeping in their stealth. Often, you will have been oblivious to or passively give way to the idea of ageing.

Looking at fellow humans performing at their peak of fitness illustrates only too clearly what most of us have come to lack. Our body's performance can drop so far below par that we simply shrug at the possibility of turning the clock back. Function may go so far awry that you acquire the companion of pain—not necessarily the raging tortured pains of broken bones, blood and gore, but aches and pains of a more subtle kind: those petty afflictions, those nuisance grumblings from our bodies that slow us down rather than stop us dead. These are not necessarily serious, but they do mean the joints and their soft tissues are subtly breaking down.

This whole bevy of afflictions commands scant regard within medical practice; they are what the medicos call 'musculo-skeletal disorders' as they dispatch us with pills and idle reassurances about 'time and rest'. These un-sexy disorders—tennis elbow, frozen shoulder, arthritis of the hip, cartilage trouble, lumbago—occur as we get older. Skeletally speaking, they are the end of the line for a joint, the final picture of acute discomfort in a slowly evolving story, when all along the way there were increasingly obvious signs from a distinctly creaking machine.

As well as these physical signs of a system seizing up, there is the cosmetic side, where we are bothered not by pain but premature ageing. That insidious cloak of debility which claims us all—if we let it—into the territory of the 'early aged'. This book is for Jo Average. Not my cyclist in the forest and not the players on centre court at Wimbledon who are out of our league. It's you I'm interested in; you who I want to bring on. I want you to do something to thwart the settling of age and, at the more ambitious, to deal successfully with unwelcome aches and pains.

What happens to the joints?

Let's assume that you are like me, the more commonplace specimen of humanity. We are the ones who momentarily catch sight of ourselves in glass shopfronts and are appalled by what we see. We have suffered the pall of time—a crook in the back or a bottom sticking out like a boomerang. Or is it our shoulders that droop or our head that is carried too far forwards, in front of the body's line of gravity? Whatever the problem, sure as eggs we think it is a sign of ageing. Our skeletons become blighted by misuse and suddenly we recognise the yoke of years.

The ultimate result of developing less than perfect muscle control is the steady loss of what is known as accessory joint movement or joint play. Joint play is best described as those intangible 'extra' movements of a joint. They are the movements between our bones which cannot be seen by the naked eye, those subtle gliding accommodating movements that give a joint an extra adaptability, an innate ability to absorb shock, a compliance that goes with being young.

A wrist joint clearly illustrates the concept of accessory movement. The wrist is not a simple hinge. It is a complex of many small bones that articulate between themselves and also with the bottom of the radius, one of the two bones of the forearm. Whatever the wrist or hand movement, there is a shuffling, harmonious interplay between all the moving parts, so the inside of the wrist resembles a bag of shuffling bones. At any point you would be hard put to say what any one bone is doing, but each is doing its own thing, in accord with the others. Rather like loose ice-cubes floating in a bag on water, every bone moves in concert but independently. This is what gives the wrist that astonishing 360-degree freedom at the bottom of the arm.

A more subtle example of accessory movement is the knee, which at face value seems to have the single action of bending and straightening. But for the knee to function optimally, it must have its full complement of internal manoeuvrability. It must be able to angle a bit, left and right, and also glide backwards and forwards, mostly to cater for irregularities in walking surfaces. More importantly, the knee must have a valuable essence of twist to bring about the complex act of locking so that we can stand on the leg without it buckling. Even from this brief description it must be obvious how un-plain the action of the knee is.

Loss of accessory movement can wreak all manner of havoc upon a joint. At best, it simply disadvantages its superlative function. At worst, it can cause crippling pain. If you suffer only minor losses of accessory movement, the joint simply loses optimum ability. It loses its quintessence of versatility, its enhanced accuracy and its ease of performance. It loses its ability to line up for that perfect angle of action. In other words, it loses its intangible quality of youth. To the senses, it has lost that 'forgiving' feel. It thuds rather than floats on air. And this is what happens as you get older. You may not realise it but under the skin the laxity is ebbing away and the joint is losing play. The subtle background movements are the first to disappear.

Of course, the ageing process is inevitable. Whatever we do or don't do, the tissues do age and become less elastic. We lose our elastin and increase our fibrin content. This means our tissues lose their ability to stretch. Just as the skin around our eyes changes and becomes wrinkled and crepey (alas!) so do the tissues around our joints, causing them to lose their bounce. They become thicker in appearance, less elastic and dry. And as the joints lose their romp, they become squeezed of their accessory movement as the margins of manoeuverability are narrowed.

But even before we get old, this process can be speeded up by poor muscle control, which puts added strain on the joints. This hastens the problems of advancing years and hard work. Returning again to the analogy of the ship's mast, it manages to stay upright while the boat floats over mirrored glassy waters. But when the going gets rough and the boat is buffeted about by waves, the extra strain will tell. If the stays haven't been looked after, the mast will eventually snap. And our joints? They are a little more enduring but without due care, they will suffer further when exposed to increased wear and tear.

It is important to understand how you can lose accessory joint freedom because of poor muscular control. Imagine the inner workings of your elbow. It operates like a double pulley, with ropes (tendons) pulling back and forth through it—one side to bend the arm, the other to straighten it. If one tendon is shorter or tighter it will chafe as it pulls through and friction will be set up between the close-knit structures. Inflammation results, with one struggling tendon less and less comfortable as it loses its capacity to accept stretch. Eventually you become more guarded, restricting movement, stopping short when you extend your elbow because going the full way invokes a stretch that hurts too much. You have unwittingly indulged the pull back, and in doing so, have relinquished an increment of the joint's freedom.

This is how it starts, and goes on. A muscle chafes, gets inflamed, and declines to stretch and a whisker of joint performance closes down. This is the early stage, though you may be unaware of what is happening. You may simply register a sore arm for a day or so, after some painting perhaps, but it goes away. You spare the joint from doing things it doesn't like. You lay off the painting and in time everything settles: inflammation soothes, swelling disperses and normality reigns. The angriness of this short-lived episode subsides but a chronic picture takes over. And here's the rub: things are not quite as normal as they were. Not quite all your joint freedom returns.

As the cloud of irritation lifts, it unveils a joint that has some compartments still closed down. If you try to push the joint where it doesn't want to go, it won't like it. At this point, you can do one of two things. Either stay as you are and don't ask the joint to do things it doesn't want to do, letting it hang onto its new tight restrictive practices, or barge on through, making the joint participate in normal activity. This latter choice can also go one of two ways. You may do just enough measured movement to coax the tight components back into full and useful function or you can go over the limit and provoke an angry reaction from the joint.

This explains why sometimes activity is right for a joint, and other times it hurts it more. Why sometimes going for a run on a sore ankle is just what it needs, but sometimes you come back hobbling. It is all to do with the degree of resistance, and getting the level of how much to push it right. Too much too fast and the joint will clam up.

This also explains how you can keep on injuring a joint— re-injuring it and injuring it again. If its performance has fallen too far below par, all your actions will amount to trauma. Anything can hurt it. The joint becomes so tight it can barely accommodate any function at all. This is common with ankles: an initial nasty wrench, then another a couple of weeks later, and thereafter the ankle is never the same again. You are always going over on it. It is always easy to hurt; basically an accident waiting to happen.

Trouble only escalates when the muscles around an injured joint lock tight. This is protective spasm, an automatic response activated when the brain senses a joint is hurt. In the case of an ankle, the muscles on all sides go so stiff it cannot be bent or straightened and you end up walking with a limp.

You may not remember when you first did something to harm a joint. You could have hurt it but just passed it off as nothing. Was it ten years ago, or maybe fifteen? You may have been vaguely aware that one joint, somehow, was not the equal of the other one. Or, you might have wondered why you keep going over on one ankle, never the other. What you didn't know was that the muscle clench had become ever-present, trimming the joint on all sides. More and more avenues of accessory joint movement had closed down. The ankle became stiffer in all different directions, setting itself up to be hurt by something as minor as treading on uneven paving stones.

This is the common picture leading up to joint injury—stealthy loss of accessory freedom. It also explains why trivial incidents can amount to major injury. 'I hardly did anything and the ankle gave way', you might say. The truth is you had it coming. The joint that was subtly and increasingly being hampered by loss of accessory freedom reached the point where any injury was going to amount to a catastrophe.

What can you do about it?

After all this bad news, you must be wondering what can be done to prevent problems or, more to the point, cure them. Well, the good news is that there is lots you can do. No matter how badly you have used your body, however improperly paired your muscle groups have become, you *can* reverse the trend. Joints can be unkinked. It is not as difficult as you might imagine and you can do it yourself at home.

To my mind, there are few things cleverer than yoga—it has all the answers. Whoever the original yogis were, they certainly knew what they were doing. They understood how joints tighten, and which movements old joints find hard to do. Accordingly, there is a complete range of yoga procedures that can be harvested for what they can do to rejuvenate each joint of your skeleton.

Yoga once had a bad name. It seemed to be associated with occult ceremonies, incense burning and breathing through one nostril. But yoga not only stretches your body it involves discipline, meditation, breathing control, elevated states of mental awareness and so on. Perhaps not all these avenues are readily accessible to the hurried habits of Westerners but each of us has something to gain from its practice. Apart from the centring and the rarified sessions of inner stillness, the supreme gift of yoga is its physical prowess; quite simply, its ability to restore accessory movement to the joints.

The fruits of yoga are plucked along the way, on the journey, not the destination. This simple tenet is readily misunderstood by yoga's dismissive band of doubters. There are also people who say, 'It hurt too much so I didn't think I should do it' or, 'I've never been able to touch my toes'. But yoga is the most simple and effective way of keeping the joints apart, of keeping them young. There is no great value in reaching the destination, no great value in reaching your toes. The value lies in the process of getting there and this is where we can get it wrong. By concentrating upon point scoring, getting the goal, end-gaining for the sake of it, we fail to appreciate the subtlety of our bodies opening out en route, the little improvements along the way, feeling looser in your own skin, feeling lighter and, yes, feeling younger.

I believe suppleness is much overlooked in today's pursuit of strength and aerobic fitness. The two are as different as night and day. Aerobic activity—say, a run, a cycle, a swim, a gym workout, or a game of squash—is the equivalent of a quick fix. You feel good at the time because of the endorphin high. But aerobic activity is a lopsided victory if you don't undo the ill-effects of accumulating strains. More importantly, it often reinforces one set of sporting patterns on top of your routine habits of movement.

Suppleness is what you want—or at least what you need. This means releasing your skeleton in myriad different directions to unhitch it from its habitual crimps and kinks. Perhaps it is our punitive work ethic that makes us see value in dripping sweat and a racing pulse. The fact that yoga takes time may turn people away, as if the qualities of calmness and deliberate anti-haste will in some way attach themselves to your working habit and rob you of the vital reserves of punch you need in your working life. Yoga is not like that.

Yoga consists of a series of unyielding edicts through exacting physical postures. But the battle is with yourself not some clock on the wall or pile of weights on a machine. It is pedantic and exacting, and the aim is to do it calmly and very well. Near enough is not good enough. You need good breathing control to make the hard things easier and, at times, it requires immense willpower to maintain lip-bitingly difficult postures. It also has to be said that many of the postures hurt.

I make it sound depressing. I make it sound as if all other forms of physical exercise are meretricious by contrast. I don't mean to (or do I?). I simply mean to extol the virtues of a subtle discipline and explain its benefits for the wider realm of health. The superiority of yoga is that it undoes our complex and often-used patterns of movement. None of the postures reinforces habitual actions and all of them reclaim forgotten territory. Unlike other forms of body stretching, yoga will undo the pattern rather than a single movement.

Yoga does take time and effort. Sometimes it is agony just to hold a stretch for a matter of seconds. But this is what it is all about. The harder you find the stretch, the more you need it. In time, all your soft tissues will loosen—even blood vessels and nerves—as the body is reintroduced to its extremes. Elasticity is restored and so is streamlined, smooth-gliding function. The stretches pull the tissues and create a much more vigorous blood supply. Blood rushes to mop up after the unexpected demands on flexibility and the circulation through the tissues changes from a torpor to a flush. The skeleton is cleansed and rejuvenated.

That leads me to the final plus of the gentle art of yoga: the staggeringly rich variety in the choice of stretches. You can start off with the most modest, disarmingly gentle stuff, where you really find it hard to believe anything is happening at all, and eventually progress to the nigh impossible. You can start at your own level and progress at any rate.

The Exercises

At the end of each of the following chapters you will find a series of yoga exercises to help restore full mobility to your joints. The exercises have been divided into beginners, intermediate and advanced and you must follow them carefully and slowly, knowing your own limits. It is better to do just a few exercises properly than rush through the whole set badly.

If you start off knowing you already have a problem, be prepared to take things slowly. At the start, it may be impossible to progress beyond the first beginners' exercise. Even then you may feel you are doing it so badly it is hardly worth continuing. But don't give up. There is nothing wrong with staying at this level for weeks if you have to. And don't worry if your efforts look nothing like the illustrations. It's all in the journey. Eventually you will get nearer to the way it looks in the book and the benefits will be happening all along the way. In the early stages, you may not be able to hold the exercise for the length of time I suggest. If this happens, come out of the posture earlier, flop your body around to ease the discomfort or even massage yourself, and then try it again.

Do not be tempted, incidentally, to try strengthening a problem joint before you have restored its full function. Whether it is a shoulder that won't go up or a knee that won't straighten, it is futile to keep exercising it to get it strong. If you approach the problem from the other direction, that is to restore its accessory performance first, you will find that the strength comes back of its own accord with minimal need for exercising.

If you do not have a specific joint problem and just need a general program, I have devised a 30-minute daily regime. It deals with all the different parts of the body in turn. As you go through, it will be apparent which joints are the most resistant to stretch. These are the areas to specifically concentrate on. Go to the chapter on that joint and do as many of these exercises as you can. This could mean an hour's workout but it is a very effective system. You will quite quickly develop your favourite exercises, just as you will sense the ones your body needs most. Hopefully these will be one and the same.

Each joint regime has been graded from the easiest to the most difficult but you should expect to do most. Even a few seconds of the hardest ones will bring results. Only in cases of severe dysfunction of a joint (discussed in each chapter under the heading 'Common dis-orders') should you be content with doing only the first couple of exercises of each regime.

If the stretches are being effective you should feel a minimal state of muscle soreness the next day, a sensation of mild but agreeable discomfort as if something is happening. If it goes beyond this and it hurts all the time then you need to lay off a bit—hold each exercise for a shorter length of time, don't do the repetition and stop short of the most demanding ones at the end of each regime. If the soreness takes more than a few days to dissipate then you should drop down to exercising twice or three times a week rather than daily. But do remember, in the overall scheme of things, soreness is no bad thing. With frank joint problems you will find the old familiar pain is replaced by a different sort of tissue tenderness. This is one of the best signs of progress.

As a rule it is better to do the stretching at the end of the day, ideally an hour or two after dinner, before going to bed. We are always stiffer in the mornings and the spectre of the looming day often makes it harder to relax your way through each exercise. Another good time is mid-morning if you are lucky enough to be home when the house is quiet and there is no rush. It is never good to do the exercise regime on a full stomach.

You must take care to keep breathing evenly as you do each exercise. Resist the temptation to hold your breath as the full discomfort of each stretch becomes apparent. Don't tense the body and fight against your own muscles. As you go into each stretch, will yourself to relax. Concentrate on slow quiet breathing and let your head float away. Use your diaphragm to suck air into your lungs from below up, creeping the air in quietly past your nasal passages without making any noise (remember, it irritates your nasal mucosa to suck air in hard through your nose). As you breathe quietly, feel the resistance of your body palpably melt as the relaxation takes effect. But as you near the limit of endurance your body will start to harden again, a sign that it is time to come out of the stretch. If you are overtired or tense, you will reach your limit sooner.

Listen to your body and watch for these subtle signs. Unclutter your mind and take it slowly, and you will be there.

Chapter one

Your low back

WHAT IS YOUR LOW BACK?

Your lumbar spine, or low back, is a short, segmented pillar that sits on the sacrum at the back of your pelvis. It works like a chunky, flexible strut that supports the rest of your spine towering above it. Your lumbar spine passes up through the back of your abdominal cavity, which balloons out in front, and a strong corseting of the abdominal muscles is required to hold your abdominal wall reefed in. Abdominal muscle weakness, common to most of us, allows the abdominal contents to fall forward, and this can have direct consequences for the functioning of your lower spine.

The lumbar spine consists of five lumbar vertebrae. The lowest, L5, is lashed securely to the forward-sloping surface of your sacrum. The sacrum does not participate in spinal mobility. It consists of five fused sacral vertebrae with the vestigial remnant of the tail, the coccyx, extending from the base. Your sacrum makes up the back wall of your pelvis and joins with the two big ear-shaped bones (the ilia) at either side at the sacro-iliac joints, the impression of which you can see as two dimples in your skin. The forward inclination of the sacrum is approximately 50 degrees. Flatter or steeper angulations of your sacrum can have direct consequences for the way your entire spine stacks, and also on the way it absorbs impact.

The vertebral body is the circular brick-like part of each vertebra. It has a narrowed waist to help bear load, though most of its weight-bearing brilliance comes from the honeycomb bone (trabeculae) on

17

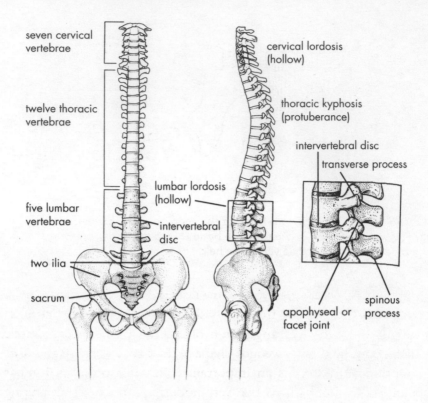

seven cervical
vertebrae

cervical lordosis
(hollow)

twelve thoracic
vertebrae

thoracic kyphosis
(protuberance)

intervertebral disc

transverse process

lumbar lordosis
(hollow)

five lumbar
vertebrae

intervertebral
disc

two ilia

sacrum

spinous
process

apophyseal or
facet joint

FIGURE 1.1 Front and side views of the human spine. The vertebral
segment is shown in close-up.

the inside of the vertebral body. All weight-bearing bones have trabeculae, which look like iron filings following lines of force, showing
where load is transmitted through the bone. These resemble the
structure of a sponge and are an ingenious way of making the bones
strong, yet light. If the vertebral bodies were solid bone, the spine
would be too heavy to lift and chunks of bone would cleave off under
load. The trabeculae form a three-dimensional grid of fine vertical
pillars and horizontal struts of bone. The vertical ones sustain load
while the horizontal ones provide transverse shoring to prevent the
vertical ones buckling. They also prevent the sides of the vertebral
body caving in like a cardboard carton.

Your lumbar spine is a bendable pillar of support. Its segments
stack around a gentle forward-arching curve known as the lumbar
lordosis, which gives your lower back a natural hollow when viewed

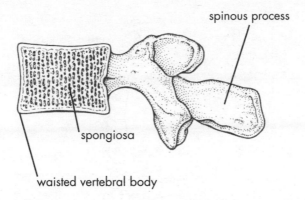

spinous process

spongiosa

waisted vertebral body

FIGURE 1.2 The honeycomb bone of the spongiosa is really a three-dimensional scaffold which stops the bone crumbling under pressure. The blood reservoirs in the vertebrae help absorb shock.

from the side. The rest of your spine uncoils in an 'S' as it rises from your pelvis, like a cobra from its basket. The lumbar spinal curve is maintained by forward angulation of your sacrum, correct muscle balance and the slightly wedged-shape back of both vertebra and disc.

Optimum lordosis is an important factor in sustaining lumbar spinal health. It performs two very important functions: a sinking and springing action on footfall, which provides a very important impact-absorbing mechanism to eliminate juddering during walking, and the more static stacking of the torso on your lower body with minimal effort, most importantly during sitting. It follows that spines with either too much or too little lumbar lordosis suffer mechanical duress. Insufficient lumbar hollowing causes added load to be borne through the front of your spine—thus loading up your discs—whereas too great a lumbar hollow causes the opposite: excessive weight-bearing through the back of your spine at the facet joints.

The intervertebral discs sit between your vertebrae like squashy water-filled pillows to cushion bone-to-bone contact. They are thickest in the lumbar area, where they provide vigorous resilience to compression. In many ways, discs resemble a radial car tyre: the walls consist of twelve to fifteen layers of diagonal meshing, the fibres of each alternate layer running at right angles to the one before. This provides great strength, yet allows the vertebrae to twist and gap open on all sides during movement.

The anulus fibrosis is the circumferential wall of the disc. It is divided into a middle-inner section plus an outer part and—very importantly—their roles are quite different. The middle-inner anulus works like a capsule, with its fibres running in a circular fashion throughout both adjacent vertebral end plates. Its fibres contain the fluid nucleus at the centre of the disc and this part is responsible for bearing load. The walls are prevented from buckling and collapsing under load by the radially 'outwards squirting' pressure of the water contained within the nuclear capsule.

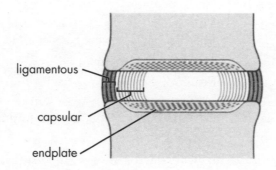

FIGURE 1.3 Anulus fibrosis (circumferential wall of an intervertebral disc).

The outer disc walls are not involved in weight bearing at all. They are more like a pre-tensioned outer ligamentous skin, which works like a connective stocking-mesh to bind the vertebral segments together. The more radially expanded the disc is by the downward force, squirting the fluid of the nucleus outwards, the more the outer walls are made taut, which gives the segment stability. It works exactly like a fully inflated inner tube of a car tyre making the outer tyre taut.

It is a beautifully ingenious mechanism. The two parts of the disc wall complement each other: the outer wall controls stretch whereas the inner controls compression. The spine then manages to combine flexibility at low load and stability at high load.

Disc hydration is the key to maintaining spinal health. A disc lacking fluid develops a lower hydrostatic pressure. It also means the walls will not be fully radially expanded, like a car tyre lacking air, and the outer walls will sag or bulge. All discs bulge more by the end of the day as they naturally lose fluid and less healthy discs bulge more readily because they have trouble holding their fluid. But moderate bulges alone are no bad thing. This is not quite the case with major disc wall prolapse over a sustained period.

In major disc prolapse, the outer disc wall can be painfully stretched, which can be a source of low back pain. It is important to note that only the outer ligamentous skin of the disc wall is innervated, meaning it behaves exactly like any other ligament of the body—it elicits pain if it is over-stretched and develops scar tissue after injury. With sustained wall prolapse (especially when a spinal segment is locked by extreme spasm of the spinal muscles) there can also be enzymatic breakdown of the wall, which means the disc will not expand again, even when the muscle spasm releases.

The watery nucleus of each disc behaves exactly like a liquid ball bearing. The compression of each spinal segment stacked vertically on its disc provides the pre-tension for each intervertebral link, thus allowing the whippy, elongated movement of the spine as a whole.

Proteoglycans is the magical x-factor of discs. It constitutes 65 per cent dry weight of the nucleii and exerts a powerful electrostatic attraction to water. Thus proteoglycans is the active osmotic agent that drags fluid into the discs, keeping them buoyantly plumped up despite the weighing down effects of gravity. Even so, fluid is gradually squeezed from the discs by day so that we all go to bed approximately 2 centimetres shorter at night. Lumbar discs lose more than those higher up because they are the cushions at the bottom of the stack. Fluid loss throughout the day is regained at night—imbibed during sleep when your body is stretched out horizontal and relaxed. The tidal exchange of discal fluids squeezed out by day and sucked back in by osmosis overnight is one of the main mechanisms of feeding your discs. If you are tense during sleep and do not relax your muscles the discs will not get back their full complement of fluid, and disc nutrition suffers. The stateliness of this diurnal fluid exchange is only tolerable because the metabolic rate of the discs is so slow. It also means that discs are only just viable, even in their normal healthy state; they are slow to break down, and also slow to repair.

A vital adjunct to the daily exchange of discal fluids is the 'pump imbibition' mechanism provided by pressure changes created by movement. This mechanism mainly works during daylight hours, when physical stretching and bending exerts a squirt–suck effect on your spinal segments, creating an ancillary circulation of discal fluids. So a full range of activities during the day keeps the discs additionally nourished. In later life, or when the discs degenerate, this secondary pump mechanism becomes more important, both to off-set reduced proteoglycans content of older discs and the calcification of small holes in the endplates, through which fluids pass to and from the vertebral bodies. At the very outset, this explains why movement is such an important factor in spinal rehabilitation—more so as you get older.

Each vertebra joins its neighbour through the vertebra–disc union, but it also makes bone-to-bone contact at the back of the bony ring. As one vertebra sits on another, they make two bony notches behind the intervertebral disc, flanking the central neural tube that houses the valuable spinal cord. These bone-to-bone notches are called the apophyseal or facet joints.

The facet joints are synovial joints like many others in the body, such as the finger joints or the knee. The facets' role is to notch the segments together in a loosely articulated column that then protects

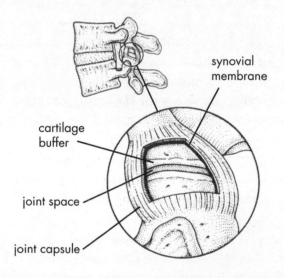

FIGURE 1.4 The opposing cartilage-covered surfaces of each facet fit together like two palms pressed together.

the central core from excessive movement, which could cause the disc walls to fray. The congruent interfaces of the facet joints are held together by their own joint capsule and their opposing cartilaginous surfaces are washed and lubricated by the supremely lightweight and slippery synovial fluid. The facet surfaces are the first to suffer rub if the washer-like disc of the same level loses water and deflates. This is another important source of lower back pain.

Like other synovial joints, the facets are strained easily and prompt pain follows. Unlike the intervertebral disc, they have a highly sophisticated nerve supply. At each intervertebral level two spinal nerves branch off the cord inside the spinal canal and issue from the column through the intervertebral foraminae. These short bony canals are situated between the segments, equidistant between the intervertebral disc at the front and the facet joint behind. Thus, the spinal nerves exit the spine right through the spinal hinges, running the gauntlet between two potential aggressors and, not surprisingly, it is fairly easy for the nerve roots to be irritated by a bulging unhealthy disc wall or an inflamed facet joint. Either condition can cause leg pain or sciatica.

HOW DOES YOUR LOW BACK WORK?

As you've just discovered, your lumbar vertebrae provide the stacking support, whereas the intervertebral discs perform the dual roles of shock absorption and gluing the cotton-reel vertebral bodies together. The facet joints steady the flamboyant column of segments by providing bone-to-bone notching, which ultimately stops them toppling off one another.

Your low back positions the thinking–acting, upper part of your body and you could say the main role of your lumbar spine is to support your upper body while letting it bend with safety through the middle.

Your spine acts as the central strut to the internal scaffolding of your body. It is tall and narrow with a handsome repertoire of movement. Bending forward is its most grandiose—and most risky—action though the combination of your spine's hard anatomy and soft tissues makes it possible.

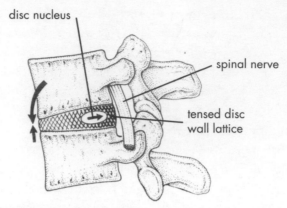

disc nucleus

spinal nerve

tensed disc
wall lattice

FIGURE 1.5 The bending action invokes its own brake when the backward migration of the nucleus makes the back wall of the disc taut; this makes it harder for the vertebrae to pull apart.

The intervertebral discs provide the dramatic cohesion between your spinal segments. They are tenaciously embedded in the flat upper and lower surfaces of their neighbouring vertebrae, and when your spine bends, their stretching outer walls steady the movement, while the thrusting, hydrostatic pressure of the nucleus helps by pre-tensioning the walls. As the vertebrae pull apart, the outer walls pull up, rather like tugging up garden lattice; the further it goes, the greater the holding tension of the mesh. When bending forwards, the strong reinforcing ligaments of the facet joints capsules—known simply as the capsular ligaments—help control the movement.

The disc walls and the capsular ligaments almost evenly share the job of holding the segments together when your spine bends, but the solid backstop to all this is the bone-to-bone notching of the facet joints. Strong as the disc walls and the capsular ligaments are, they would eventually fray and weaken were it not for the bony inter-lock of the spinal facets.

Your facet joints are the ultimate block to your spine coming undone. Their upper and lower joint surfaces notch together to prevent shear. It's a bit like locking the hands by cupping the finger-tips over each other. You can see the effectiveness of this facet chain in the dry bones of a cadaver (minus the discs). They stack upright fairly securely, the mutual bony surfaces butting against each other, and don't fall apart until the spine is well advanced in a forward lean.

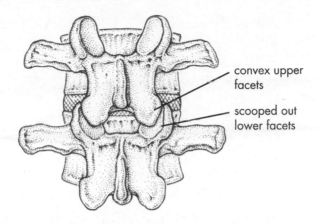

convex upper
facets

scooped out
lower facets

FIGURE 1.6 The cupped bowl of the lower facet surfaces notches the vertebrae together and facilitates forward bending only.

In the living, the soft tissues of the spine—mainly the discs and the facet capsules—prevent the segments coming apart in this way.

Quite apart from being useful, bending has an important role to play in keeping intervertebral discs healthy. Discs do not have a blood supply; they are the largest avascular structure in the body. They require movement of fluids to take in raw materials—particularly the larger molecules—and expel waste products. High fluid content and a robust fluid exchange is the mainstay of disc nutrition and a healthy back. Disc health is all about disc hydration.

Proteoglycans exerts an osmotic pull on water and is a vital essence in disc hydration. A higher concentration of proteoglycans keeps discs better hydrated and degenerated discs have a lower percentage of proteoglycans. Sick discs have trouble holding their water. The synthesis of proteoglycans is stimulated by pressure changes within the discs—and the optimum range is between 0.3 and 2.5 megapascals (MPa). This just happens to be within physiological range—2.5 megapascals is the maximum pressure recorded when lifting a 20-kilogram weight.

Pressure changes are vitally important to the health of discs and for this reason it is essential for spines to move—indeed to lift—to remain healthy. On the other hand, synthesis of proteoglycans declines when discs endure sustained pressures, either high or low.

This explains why bed rest is not good for recuperating spines, nor is sustained sitting. Both extremes are not good for disc vitality.

Degeneration of a spinal segment usually happens via the two main mechanisms that hold the segment together—the disc or the facet capsule. Disc drying and thinning is usually the primary process.

As a disc desiccates from spinal compression, its segment becomes stiff and painful in the column. I call this the stiff spinal segment (Stage 1) and believe it is the most likely cause of simple lower back pain. As the disc degenerates and loses hydrostatic pressure, its walls bunch down and the segment loses mobility. Eventually this implicates the facets at the same level, which also lose mobility as the facet capsules become tighter. This puts them next in line in suffering strain and the ensuing inflammations is known as facet joint arthropathy (Stage 2). As the disc becomes distinctly thinner, the facets start to bear load and their bone-to-bone interfaces become eroded and bruised, resulting in frank arthritic degeneration of the facet joints. As a degenerated disc struggles to hold its water its walls distend, like a half-deflated car tyre; more so at the end of the day. Disc walls bulge even further if the segment is locked up by protective muscle spasm. This may be seen with CT and MRI scanning but may be misinterpreted as disc prolapse.

Acute facet locking (Stage 3) happens when a small unguarded movement causes a facet to slightly slip askew as a consequence of early disc thinning and reduced intra-discal pressure. Instantaneously, your spine will lock up in an agonising gust of protective spasm, which can take weeks to dissipate. This fluke mishap is often memorable many years later and can mark your spine's downfall; the point beyond which it was never the same again.

Alternatively, the segment may go the other more insidious route where low-grade muscle spasm keeps a spinal link pinched in the column. If a disc wall has been buckled and flat for too long, it will be attacked by enzymatic action, like a car tyre perishing as it runs along almost on the rim. After several weeks like this, the disc cannot be rehydrated and the disc bulge becomes permanent, even when the muscle spasm comes off. This is true intervertebral disc prolapse (Stage 4), although it is often diagnosed in error. Disc prolapse is not a common cause of back (or leg) pain.

Once discs degenerate beyond a certain point, they can no longer hold their segments together firmly in the column and they tend to ooze forward under sustained spinal compression. Over time, this recurrent trespass weakens the other main stabilising structures of the segment: the capsular ligaments or the capsules of the facet joints. Eventually, there is a noticeable forward slippage of this segment every time the spine goes to bend. This condition is known as 'segmental instability' and it manifests as a weak back with a painful catch when the spine goes forward. It can also manifest as the spine giving way, or simply as a painful arc on bending (Stage 5).

The trend with segmental breakdown is for a normal segment to become stiff, then unstable, though few cases progress right through to instability. A stiff spinal segment is the most common cause of lower back pain (up to 90 per cent of cases). This progression of breakdown is discussed in greater detail in another of my books, *The Back Sufferers' Bible*.

Muscle control plays an important role in segmental stability and the way your spine moves as a whole. Both your tummy muscles (abdominals) at the front of your spine and your deep spinal muscles (intrinsics) at the back, control segmental mobility. Working as a group, the layers of tummy muscles—superficial, intermediate and deep—perform two functions: first, as a retaining wall and, second, offloading the spine to prevent segmental compression. The oblique muscles (of the intermediate layer) and the transversus abdominus (of the deep) play a significant role in stabilising your spinal segments.

A strong abdominal wall reduces the ever-present weighing-down effects of gravity. In offloading some of the compression on the lower spinal segments it thwarts breakdown of your lumbar discs. It does this by tightening your girth, pulling your tummy in like a grey-hound's, which then pressurises and elongates the intra-abdominal space. A reefing-in contraction of these hoists up your spine (and the abdominal contents), in the same way that grasping an open plastic bottle of water causes water to spurt out the top.

Abdominal muscles also help with bending. They work like a retaining wall at the front, with abdominal back-pressure preventing forward shear of the segments as your spine leans over. The internal and external oblique muscles and the transversus abdominus work differently. They circle your abdomen transversely and anchor into a diagonal mesh called the lateral raphe, which in turn attaches to the sides of your lumbar vertebrae. As they contract they pull the lattice out transversely, which shrinks it vertically. This telescopes your spinal segments down on to one another and makes them more secure as your spine bends. The transversus abdominus works in tandem with the very important intrinsic muscles at the back of your spine (multifidus), which attach to the individual vertebrae.

Both tranversus abdominus and intrinsic muscles work directly on the spinal segments during bending. They attach in a variety of directions—vertically, horizontally and diagonally—to the fin-like bony extensions projecting from the sides and back of each vertebrae. They steady bending by 'paying out' to their length and letting their vertebrae gape apart at the back to tip, glide or swivel in a controlled way.

Their dynamic influence on spinal stability is put to good use in the rehabilitation of segmental instability. Re-educating intrinsic strength helps compensate for laxity of trans-segmental ligaments— including a flaccid disc—and thus helps overcome the tendency of a vertebra to shear forward during bending.

Intrinsics strengthening can make all the difference as to whether a loose segment needs surgical stabilisation by spinal fusion. A seemingly small contribution of volitional control from the tranversus abdominus plus the intrinsics makes all the difference to ease of bending, and can eradicate a swerving painful arc of movement, so typical of instability. Powerful unfurling exercises off the end of a table can provide the strength for muscles to control their individual vertebra; converting the trunk into a strong, bendable pillar, where previously it may have folded up like a broken reed whenever it left the safety of vertical.

WHAT ARE THE ACCESSORY MOVEMENTS OF YOUR LOW BACK?

Inter-segmental freedom is the vital accessory movement of the spine. These are the incremental movements of the vertebrae; each one making its virtuoso effort towards grand spinal movement, like individual members of an orchestra contributing to a symphony. Vertebral distraction (separation) is the most important accessory movement, although this is not brought about by muscle effort. It is the product of all the other accessory freedoms. Vertebral distraction is significant because it is the converse of segmental compression.

Bending forward is our most important functional activity. The degree of forward movement of individual vertebrae is small but superimposed, vertebra on vertebra, the overall range of the spine as a whole is phenomenal. With one flourishing move you can stoop to get wet clothes from a washing basket, and then arch back fully, arms aloft, to peg them to the line. In contrast, any man-made device would be heavy and cumbersome, with pulleys and counterweights to control what the back does silently and compactly under the skin.

When you bend your spine forward, there is an incremental slide of upper on lower vertebrae and then, as they start to tip, a gap opens up at the back. The interspace opening at the back disengages the facets so the top vertebra can glide forward some more. This small increment of forward glide adds a profound extra dimension to your overall range of spinal movement, ensuring your upper vertebra is positioned slightly forward to the one below before it starts to do its own thing. If there were no forward glide and the vertebrae remained stacked directly over one another, your range of movement would be a fraction of what it is.

Segmental glide is the secret to effortless spinal movement. But more importantly, it keeps your discs elastic so the segments are free to pull apart. Keeping the walls stretchable introduces valuable pressure changes through your discs, which are necessary for stimulating proteoglycans synthesis. Distraction of the spinal segments also allows your discs to actively suck in fluid to keep themselves plumped up. Stretchable walls mean your discs are freer to imbibe fluid when you are passively horizontal overnight. Remember that healthy nuclear material will attempt to swell by up to 300 per cent, but it cannot do this if your disc walls are too stiff to allow each disc to take in water and grow.

Important as accessory movements are, it is really the hidden element of segmental separation that is critical. Segmental separation per se cannot be felt by a manual therapist. Rather it is the other freedoms of forward glide (thumbs on the back of the spinous process) or swivel (pressures transversely against the spinous process) that indicate if separation will be there too. The main focus of manual therapy to your spine is seeking out and restoring these small components of accessory movement. Forward glide is the most sought after, simply because it has the most potential to provide vertebral separation.

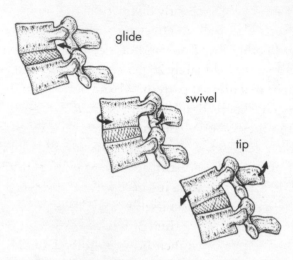

FIGURE 1.7 All the vertebrae glide, swivel and tip to a small degree, but together, overall spinal movement is grandiose.

Vertebral glide is what we manual therapists spend a lifetime looking for. We feel around in human spines, and when we encounter lack of glide we say the vertebra is stiff or jammed. As you lie prone, your low back slack and relaxed over a pillow, it is surprising how easy it is to feel degrees of segmental freedom. Rather like tinkering with piano keys, the stiff ones are immediately apparent because they are hard to depress, and any stiffness is usually matched by your pain. A stiff vertebra feels sore when touched as if the bone itself is bruised.

Segments may be free to glide some ways but not others. A segment may go forwards, for example, or swivel when pushed to the right, but it may be completely blocked from the left, or vice versa. Blockage of glide, even if isolated to one vertebral level, and one freedom at that level, still constitutes a function fault in overall spinal mobility. It will still peg down the walls of a disc so its nucleus cannot take in fluid and puff up. And remember, a dry leaden shock absorber disc is the first flaw.

HOW DOES YOUR LOW BACK GO WRONG?

Generally speaking, two background factors cause breakdown of your low back: the long-term impaction of the base due to gravity, and abnormal spinal curvatures. Both diminish accessory movement of the lumbar segments, particularly distraction.

Gravity exerts a squashing effect on your spine, more so at the lower end, like compressing one end of a concertina. Each day, your lumbar discs lose approximately 20 per cent of their fluid, which they retrieve at night in a diurnal pattern. When you wake in the morning your discs are chockablock full of fluid and they gradually deflate as you get up and move about. This may be the cause of early morning stiffness, which gets easier as the day goes on and the discs start emptying. If your back gets stiff again at the end of the day the reasons are different; this time it's because the bony segments meet as the spine telescopes down on itself when the discs deflate.

This slow tidal exchange of fluid provides nutrition and disc maintenance, and in keeping with their heavy workload, lumbar discs lose and gain more than other parts of the spine. Full-range spinal activity during daylight hours performs two basic tasks: first, it keeps the disc walls elastic so they are stretchy enough to accommodate the full quota of return fluid each night and, second, it sucks small quantities of fluid in through the day to retard disc flattening. This has important ramifications for spinal health, as it does obviously for rehabilitation programs.

The two systems of discal fluid exchange complement each other if you lead a normal, active life. If you keep the discs mobile, you recoup at night exactly the same amount of fluid you lost throughout the day. Discs lose up to 10 per cent—exactly half their daily loss—in the first two hours of sitting, which allows your lumbar vertebrae to settle into closer contact. Trouble sets in for your low back if you don't bend and move enough to give your discs a drink, or if you sit for too long. Both milk the discs faster. The sustained high pressures of sitting also depress cellular activity of your discs.

Although bending properly flies in the face of conventional wisdom, it should be only too clear how important it is. Bending (right down to the toes) is beneficial in many important ways: it creates pressure changes through your discs, which stimulates their metabolism; it physically sucks fluid in and retards flattening; it keeps the tough rim of the disc wall fully elastic; it prevents tightening (contracture) of the powerful capsular ligaments of the facets; it keeps your spinal intrinsic muscles strong; and it prevents your spinal cord and its nerve roots from becoming tethered inside the spinal canal. It should be obvious what a crime it is not to bend if your back is bad. Bear in mind though, you do need strong tummy muscles to bend with safety.

With optimal antero–posterior (front–back) alignment of your lumbar (vertebrae) in the standing position, most axial load is taken through the discs at the front of your spine. Only 16 per cent of load should be taken by the facet joints at the back of the segment. As the disc of a stiff spinal segment dries out and drops in height the facet joints are the next to suffer. As the disc loses water, the upper vertebra settles down closer to the one below. This causes the bony interfaces of the facet joints to override, rather like letting a tyre down makes it ride along on the rim. With marked disc thinning the facet joints may bear up to 70 per cent of the load through the segment. These delicate joints are not designed to bear weight and inflammation is the direct consequence.

When your lower back has too great a hollow (i.e. it is hyper-lordotic) the lower lumbar facets may become a major source of pain. When your sacrum is tilted forward more than 50 degrees it encourages your spine to slide forward, down the sacral table. This causes your lumbo-sacral facets (where the spine sits on the sacrum) to permanently engage to stop the slippage. Thus, they shoulder greater than 16 per cent of load. And from here, even a slight drop in disc height can make the jamming greater. The cartilage that covers the opposing facet joint surfaces is abraded by the grinding contact. The joint capsule becomes puffy and swollen as its synovial lining secretes more fluid to sluice the joint free of the rasped-off fragments of cartilage.

Weak abdominal muscles can also allow your pelvis to tip forward and the lumbar spine to hang on its facets. This can account for the pain of a typical beer-belly posture and also that of late-stage pregnancy. It is the most readily reversible cause of lower back pain, with pain modifying within days of an abdominal strengthening regime starting.

With a too-straight or humped lower back the discs take the brunt of axial load and the facets little or nil. A humped lower back also means the lower back absorbs impact poorly during walking. When your spine cannot momentarily sink into a deeper lumbar hollow on heel-strike it will suffer greater duress (more so with running). If it meets the ground like a semi-straight pogo-stick your lumbar segments cannot squelch forward to ride out the compression. Over time, this incessant ramming-down telescoping of your spinal segments takes its toll. With each step, your lumbar segments thud on their disc walls, and without sufficient oomph in the deflated nucleus to spring the vertebra up again, your spine does not ride well. It is easy to see how something as simple as a poor lumbar lordosis is a potent reason for lower back problems hanging on.

In truth, the discs themselves receive the initial brunt of trauma but, as you will see later, disc thinning and degeneration is an important first step in the breakdown of a spinal segment. As the disc thins, overloading of the facets makes them next in line.

Sitting creates a much higher intra-discal pressure, caused by the pelvis ramming up under the descending column, and this causes faster fluid loss from lumbar discs. Degenerated discs lose their water more readily since they have a lower concentration of proteoglycans. Faulty sitting can make matters worse. If the entire length of your spine slumps in a 'C' shape instead of keeping an ideal 'S' bend, where the lower back retains a hollow, you exert an even greater squashing pressure on your lower discs. Very little weight is shared by the facet joints at the back, and the cotton reel-shaped bodies of the vertebrae bear down on one another at the front, pressing fluid out of their discs even faster.

With static sitting, axial load is transferred from the nucleus to the disc walls. Extended periods of sitting on the disc walls causes them to become fibrotic and less able to pull apart and rehydrate when the pressure comes off. To compound matters, the sustained loading reduces the metabolic rate of the lumbar discs and slows disc cell synthesis. In this way, the lumbar discs become starved of fluid and permanently thinner. Your lower back is then set up for trouble: the more compressed your spine is, the less it can absorb incidental shock and the more susceptible it is to future injury.

This can be compounded by the general stoop of your skeleton during everyday activity. With a habitual mode of concentration, your frame will curl forwards to focus your eyes over a small field of vision (threading a needle, putting a key in the door, moving a cursor on a computer screen), which causes your skeleton as a whole to lose its ability to arch backwards, while at the same time your lower spine becomes trapped in a rigid hoop.

A tethered-over posture disturbs the background 'balance of freedom' of your whole skeleton. Its poor dynamic balance means that key load-bearing points of your skeleton—your shoulders, hips, both ends of the spine—slowly accumulate strain and cause you all sorts of aches and pains. Seemingly out of the blue you may suffer a paralysing pain in the side of your neck as you lift your head off the pillow, or your shoulder grates getting on your coat. The truth is you had it coming; problems were brewing under the surface, perhaps all of your upright life. None of the body's joints work well when your skeleton is not balanced and well-aligned.

A scoliotic lumbar spine causes low back pain from both jammed spinal segments and facet arthropathy. A scoliosis is a lateral buckling through your spine when viewed from behind and it is often caused by unequal leg lengths. A lateral curvature in your lumbar spine may be concave to the right or left and this is usually considered to be primary, and a concavity in the opposite direction, higher up the spine, is secondary. It is common—though by no means universal—that the lumbar spine's concavity will occur to the side of a longer leg

As your spine bends sideways, its stretches the sides of the discs on the convex side and pinches them together in the concavity, with the segment at the apex of the curve the most caught. The stretch and compression of both sides of the disc wall also stiffens the discs and causes several spinal segments to lose mobility. Disc cellular activity lessens on the pinched concave side of the apical disc, thus escalating that disc's breakdown. The segment at the apex of a spinal curve is always the stiffest.

Throughout a scoliotic curvature, spinal segments twist on their axes as they bend sideways. This causes facet joints to be pulled open on one side and pressed shut on the other. Altered mechanical forces from one longer leg will eventually cause facets to remould

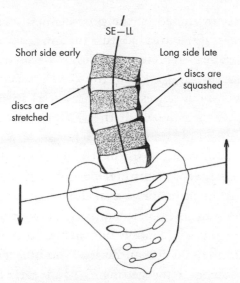

FIGURE 1.8 Back pain tends to occur on the side of the shorter leg in younger years and the side of the longer leg later in life.

their shape, though this can also result in tropism, or developmental asymmetry in facet orientation. Bearing in mind that the role of facets is to act as door stops to prevent rotation, it should be no surprise that tropism can lead directly to disc degeneration through excessive torsion strains suffered by the discs. In reality, there is a 90 per cent correlation between facet asymmetry and lower back pain. As a general rule, pain on the longer leg side tends to come on in later life, while the side of the shorter leg causes pain in the younger years.

THE COMMON DISORDERS OF THE LOW BACK

A stiff spinal segment

A compressed and brittle column of spinal segments is an easy target to shock. A lifting incident often marks the beginning of a back problem, but it can be something much more trivial, like tripping on a paving stone or turning over in bed. A jolt may penetrate the side flank of your spine, where the protective ligaments are weaker. Whichever way it comes, a yanking strain can easily stress a drier disc when its sensitive outer walls are too stiff to ride out the shock. Fibres of the ligamentous outer disc wall are stretched and broken and, though the disc is largely bloodless, there is microscopic oozing of traumatic exudate (fluid) around the site of damage in the wall.

As the torn area heals it forms scar tissue, which makes the disc walls stiffer and even less elastic during future movement. As the disc loses ability to pull apart, it houses less water and drops further in height. Eventually the diagonal fibres of the compressed wall gum together, making the disc like a hardened washer between its two vertebrae, which is resistant to stretch. Your vertebra cannot participate and pull apart with its neighbours as your spine moves.

This is the most likely cause of a stiff spinal segment, where no postural anomalies exist. The problem vertebra feels stiff and hard when manually pressured to glide forward but it may also resist lateral pressure, through the spinous process, to swivel on its axis. The problem segment becomes like a stiff link in a bicycle chain and the cycle of trauma escalates as it cannot roll with the punches and stiffness builds on stiffness.

Muscle spasm is an automatic response to protect the tender segment and reduce its demands of movement. Your back becomes armour-plated and painful as the sore link is locked away. Fear can escalate the problem and make the spasm worse. Treatment usually requires muscle-relaxant drugs in combination with rocking the knees to the chest to get all original movement back; otherwise

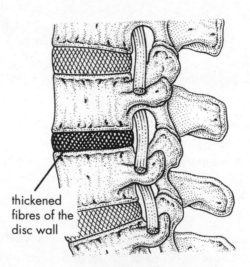

thickened fibres of the disc wall

FIGURE 1.9 A narrower disc of a stiff spinal segment.

you will be left with a much stiffer (and more painful) link. If muscle spasm takes hold and gets out of control it can make a stiff segment dramatically worse.

Stiffness of a spinal segment—usually of L5, the bottom vertebra, but also of L4 and L3, the next two up—is by far the commonest cause of simple lower back pain. In its acute form, it can be sickeningly painful, with even the lightest pressure on your back unbearable. It may be difficult for you to remain standing though it may be possible to get relief by pressing the sacrum back into a wall (which provides slight traction). By the end of the day, it is often a race against time for a mother to get dinner on the table before having to lie down. The pain can often be accurately pinpointed to a specific level and can feel like a hot coal in the back. Patients often wonder if they have cancer.

Objectively the back can feel puffy, as if the tissues are waterlogged and the segments seem squashed together. They often feel bunched together and sitting up proud, like beads threaded too tightly on elastic. Though exquisitely tender, superficially to manual palpation, deeper pressures to glide the vertebra deeper into range are often less painful. For this reason, I often use heel pressures on the spine in a treatment program.

In its more chronic form, the pain of stiff spinal segments is a diffuse centralised backache. It can radiate to the sides (high lumbar) or into both buttocks (lower lumbar), although it can be more one-sided, paraspinal, if there is loss of accessory one-way axial twist of the problem vertebra. Typically, a stiff segment feels locally sore with a bruised tenderness of the bony knob on direct pressure, as if it has been hit with a hammer. Degrees of objective stiffness can vary from a barely discernable blockage in the one-way freedom of the vertebra, to rigid immobility where the lower lumbar segments feel gnarled and rock-hard, like stuck together corroded bolts.

Facet joint arthropathy

Unlike the discs, facet joints have a sophisticated nerve supply and the sources of lower back pain, when they are inflamed, can be multiple. In addition to the deep ache beside your spine from the bony rubbing of the facet surfaces, the bloated tension of the trapped synovial fluid stretching the facet capsule can cause a sharper knife-like pain. A swollen facet joint can be felt under the skin a few centimetres out from your spine. It typically craves pummelling local pressure (with your own thumbs or knuckles) to gain relief.

Because the facet joint and its capsule are so vascular (rich in blood), acute facet arthropathy typically presents as a savage sciatic pain. It is usually described as a hot wave of pins and needles that floods down the leg when the swollen joint is pinched. Symptoms stem from the inflamed spinal nerve, by virtue of its close proximity to both the angry facet joint and swollen joint capsule. Manual pressure to the capsule often heightens the leg pain, thus making it possible to distinguish between facet joint sciatica and that of disc prolapse.

The inflammation makes the capsule feel like a tense ping pong ball under the muscles to the side of the spine. Manual contact causes a shrill pain locally, though it quite quickly evacuates the joint, as if it is being milked. By comparison, the feel of a healthy facet joint is empty when probing fingers encounter no resistance. Familiar pain can often be elicited by bending towards the side of pain, which squashes the bloated joint.

Facet joint arthropathy in its more chronic (subdued) form can cause more widespread and low-key pain in the side of the back and also further afield in the haunch and leg. Referred pain is not the same as direct inflammation of the nerve and arises when structures sharing the same nerve supply as the problem joint mistakenly feel pain. Depending on the level of the problem facet joint, pain can be felt over the iliac crest (L1–2), the hip and front of the thigh (L3), the side of the thigh and front of the shin (L4), the back of the thigh and calf (L5), and the foot (L5–S1), though distribution varies somewhat from one person to the next.

In addition to pain, there may be other symptoms of discomfort in your leg which are difficult to put a name to. Certain parts of your leg may feel increased sensitivity, as if the buttock is bonier, or the nerves in the leg are nearer the surface. Your leg can feel numb, your foot cold, or your leg have a prickling sensation as if ants are crawling over it, or the skin feels wet. Sometimes the leg simply feels heavier and

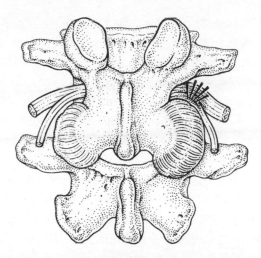

FIGURE 1.10 Pain from facet arthropathy can be referred from the inflamed joint or from direct imflammation of the nerve root.

not quite part of the body. This can all be attributed to mechanical dysfunction and inflammation of a facet joint causing disturbed neural function. At the same time, the facet itself will feel leathery and thickened under the skin, with discomfort brought on by leaning away and stretching the problem facet.

Acute locked back

Insidious loss of disc height can lead to problems when the reduced intradiscal pressure cannot spring-load its vertebra, which comes to light when the spine makes a small movement. As your spine goes to bend, in what is often seen as an inconsequential movement, such as leaning forward to pick up a coffee cup, your life can be brought to a halt in one defining moment. A wracking jolt of pain, like an electric shock through your back, can bring you to your knees as your body sets seemingly in stone.

When the juicy wedge of disc between the two vertebrae shrivels, the segment is not as well sprung apart to resist wobble as the spine bends. With reduced tensile strength, the onus is on the facets (both the bone-against-bone block and the strong capsular ligaments) to control incremental movement of the top vertebra on the bottom.

Mostly, the facets at the same level hold well enough and the disc's incompetence is not put to the test. But if your luck is out—and more particularly if you fail to brace the tummy to prime the disc—a facet joint can come undone, as its opposing surfaces slip askew. With a great punching gust your trunk muscles will seize in an instantaneous protective spasm, which freezes you part-way through a movement. You can't go up or down and you can take, literally, hours to crawl to the telephone.

Some people do manage to get to the hospital by ambulance, and the best course of action is an injection of painkillers and muscle relaxants and to go home to bed for several days. As the medication takes effect you need to move early to work the jammed facet free (rocking the knees to your chest) but tummy strengthening, particularly of the deepest muscle layer, also needs to start soon after. Reverse curl ups (bringing the knees up to your chin while the head stays flat on the floor) must be started soon to improve your core stability. In particular, you must strengthen the important transversus abdominus muscle, the specific role of which is to switch on a split second before your trunk starts to bend, to clench the lumbar segments vertically. This stops your spine coming undone as your body goes to move. Later on, after the acute phase has passed, you will need to

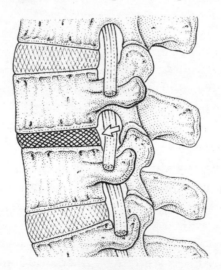

FIGURE 1.11 Minute subluxation of a facet may have its provenance in a drier, depressurised disc at the same level.

perform spinal decompression techniques to puff up the flattened disc, which is the root cause of the problem.

A 'slipped' disc

As a disc progressively thins and loses pressure, the lack of buoyancy of the nucleus means the disc walls take the brunt of the load bearing down through your spine. With a disc's poor internal squirting pressures, the meshed disc wall suffers pulverising compression, rather like resting a concrete slab on top of a wicker basket. As degeneration proceeds, the weakened nucleus loses cohesion and butts up against the inner layers of the disc wall every time your spine takes weight and the segment is flattened. The increasingly traumatised disc wall develops internal radial cracks, which the runaway nucleus burrows into from the inside out. Intense local protective muscle spasm can greatly add to the compression on the sick disc. A tense focal bulge pushes out the disc wall. When the disc has been crumpled and compressed for some time, enzymatic action attacks the wall and makes the disc's return to normal health impossible.

Your spinal nerve root can be stretched (and inflamed) as it passes by the ballooning side of the disc wall on its way out of your spine. This manifests as a deep-seated, cramping ache in your leg, made worse by any effort to move your leg forward, which stretches the nerve. Even lying on your back and raising your straightened leg off the bed by a few centimetres can bring on excruciating pain. You may feel numbness and muscle weakness in your leg or foot, depending on which fibres in the spinal nerve are being irritated. If you can stand at all, you must bend the bad leg to take weight off the disc and the tension off the nerve.

Your trunk may be thrown out of alignment by the unequal contraction of the paraspinal muscles creating the typical 'windswept' look of sciatic scoliosis, where one hip protrudes out to one side. The condition takes months to subside since nervous tissue is so unforgiving once it has been irritated. Once again, movement is the therapy, to slowly improve disc nutrition and stimulate the synthesis disc cell metabolism. Disc regeneration is slow but possible and infinitely preferable to surgical removal.

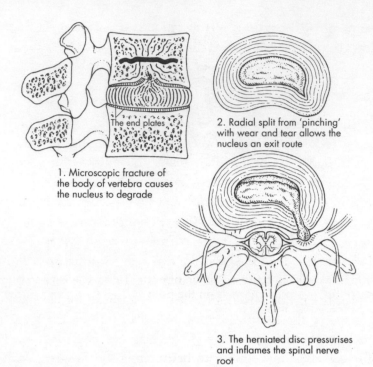

1. Microscopic fracture of the body of vertebra causes the nucleus to degrade

The end plates

2. Radial split from 'pinching' with wear and tear allows the nucleus an exit route

3. The herniated disc pressurises and inflames the spinal nerve root

FIGURE 1.12 Primary disc leads to disc prolapse.

Segmental instability

Segmental instability occurs when a spinal segment becomes wobbly in the spinal chain. It is the end-condition in the breakdown of a segment, when it changes from being stiff to loose. The instability comes to light as your spine bends forward (its most precarious movement), when the segment goes to slip. In reality, the subtle accessory vertebral movement of forward glide becomes excessive and turns into forward shear.

Although true segmental instability is uncommon, it comes about with the breakdown of the two structures that hold a spinal segment together—the intervertebral disc and the facet joints. Instability develops slowly. The symptoms gradually change from gnawing stiffness, which may have caused years of grumbling trouble, to a back that gives way under pressure. In the route of breakdown, you may pass through the phases of stiff spinal segment, facet joint arthropathy, acute locked back and disc prolapse, or you may leapfrog and go straight from a stiff segment to an unstable one.

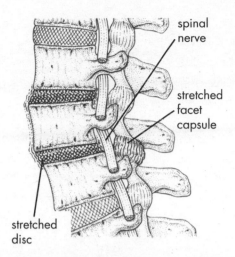

spinal
nerve

stretched
facet
capsule

stretched
disc

FIGURE 1.13 When the fibrous union of both disc and facets becomes stretched, the segment must rely on the primitive bony notching of the facets to keep itself in place.

The process is more likely to be initiated by the disc, since disc degeneration and thinning is commonplace. In the early stages your spine will develop a slight wriggle with bending, as a way of going around the weak link, but as it gets more advanced your spine can fold up like a broken reed as soon as it leaves the safety of vertical.

The specific lack of pressure in the ailing nucleus brings the characteristic wriggle to the fore; though for years the immobility of the segment may have masked its weakness and kept the segment safe (though painful). At the end of the line, the non-buoyant disc cannot act as an adequate fulcrum to spring-load its vertebra to tip it as the spine bends over. So instead, the vertebra slews forward on the flaccid disc and the runaway movement stretches the restraining structures.

For all its weakness, the loose vertebra is often completely smothered by over-protective spinal muscles, so an unstable back often feels extraordinarily stiff and painful: the so-called ironing board back. The stiffness may extend up into the thoracic spine, and indeed cause many of its symptoms there. Most commonly, though, the condition presents with pain in your leg, which may swap from side to side. This condition is often misdiagnosed as a prolapsed intervertebral disc.

The definitive symptoms of segmental instability are a sense of weakness in your back and a feeling of giving way on bending forward—typically when you lean over the hand basin in the morning—and also a wriggle or tendency to veer off to the side, instead of going straight over when bending forward. The back may click during certain actions and may get stuck turning over in bed. The telltale signs of instability are bony outgrowths (exostoses) or teeth developed at the inter-body joint, which can be seen on X-rays.

Early treatment concentrates on relaxing the over-protective long spinal muscles, which inadvertently adds greater compression on the sick disc. In the acute stage, the best exercises are rocking your knees to your chest and rolling along your spine, both of which switch off over-active paraspinals. Later, treatment must include strengthening your deep tummy muscles (reverse curl ups) and your small intrinsic muscles, which pass from vertebra to vertebra (toe touching and slowly unfurling to vertical). These two exercises help tie the loose link tighter in the column.

Once again, the most important issue (and the raison d'être of this book) is dealing with the root cause of your lower back problems: decompressing the spinal base and attempting to get more fluid into a sick and flattened disc. Segmental instability that is resistant to conservative management may need surgical fusion.

WHAT CAN YOU DO ABOUT IT?

The best way to thwart the inexorable degenerative process is to keep your spine free from the effects of impaction. The fundamental accessory movement to recapture is passive elongation (distraction) of your spine. If you can achieve this you will interrupt spinal breakdown.

Remember, we all sit too much (the national, no, international pastime) and we all stoop forward to concentrate. This directs us all towards lower back trouble. At the very least, spinal elongation prevents back problems and at its best it can help cure one—even a sinister one. If you get used to decompressing your spine, as a way of life, you can thwart the inevitable progression of the chain of events just described.

Believe it or not, it is not actually important what is wrong with your lower back—disc or facet, or a combination of the two—they all benefit from the reversal of ever-present compression. The BackBlock procedure as outlined on page 51 not only separates your lumbar vertebrae but unkinks your entire frame, taking it out of its habitual hoop and realigning the set of your skeleton. For maximum benefit, use it in the evenings when your spine is most compressed.

Beginners

Knees rocking

This universal panacea exercise is particularly important if you have just hurt your back. It uses the thighs as leverage to open and close the backs of the spinal interspaces and the pumping action evacuates stale blood and swelling collected around the facet joints so that your back should be less sore. You can do the movement for up to 5 minutes if necessary, but always bearing in mind that less is more; the muscles relax more if the movement amplitude is less. If it is effective, it should make you feel so sleepy it will be difficult to keep awake. Your back will be relaxing by the minute and your head will feel like it is floating away. You will need to repeat the exercise every 2 hours throughout the day and evening for the most benefit.

1   Lie on your back on a folded towel on a carpeted floor.
2   Bring your right knee up to your chest and hold it with your right hand, then bring up the left knee and hold with your left hand.

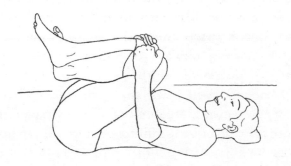

3 Spread your knees as wide apart as is comfortable, still cupping them with your hands, and cross your ankles.
4 Oscillate your legs to your chest with your head relaxed on the floor. Do not tug at the knees causing the muscles of your neck to stand out. Feel your lower spinal interspaces opening at the back as your bottom gradually lifts further off the floor. You may alternate between rocking the knees up and down, then left to right and then in small circles, first clockwise then anti-clockwise
5 Continue for up to 5 minutes and repeat the exercise 2 hours later.

Rolling along the spine

Although this exercise seems facile it is very complicated in a neurophysiological sense. As you tip forward the tummy muscles are activated and as you come back up the back muscles do their work. Rolling up and down effectively breaks up the domination of the overactive long spinal muscles and the corresponding reflex inhibition of your tummy muscles. In effect, spinal rolling halts the status quo of the back muscles not being switched off and the tummy not switched on.

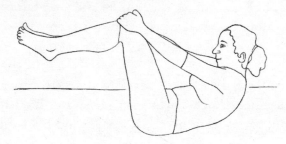

1 Lie on your back on a folded-over towel on a soft carpeted floor.
2 Lift your arms off the floor, stretching them out, and bring your thighs up so that they are just below vertical (to the floor).
3 Make your back into a round saucer-shape, tucking your chin into your chest.
4 Tip gently back and forth along the spine with very small amplitude rocking movements. Attempt to focus on the painful vertebra, as if you are pivoting on a painful cog in a wheel. This can be hard work for the tummy (and also the front of the neck) but if the going

is easy you can alternate between tipping up and down the spine to tipping left to right, pivoting on the painful vertebra.

5 To localise the lower lumbar vertebrae (L4, L5), bring your thighs slightly lower. To isolate the high lumbar and lower thoracic area, straighten the legs, holding the toes (if possible) or behind the knees.

Child's pose

This is the gentlest way to start spinal decompression through segmental separation. This posture primarily opens the facet joints at the back of the spinal interspaces and stretches the capsular ligaments, which are so strong they tend to lose elasticity easily. It is the least threatening spinal bending exercise and ideal to start with if you have not bent your back properly for years. If your knees are painful you can place a pillow on the calves to perch your bottom on.

1 On your knees, lie the tops of your feet flat on the floor then sit on your heels.
2 Separate your knees slightly and lean forward to rest your belly snugly between your thighs, lowering your upper body towards the floor. If possible rest your forehead on the floor.

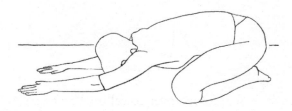

3 To add stretch, take your arms out to the front, stretching them along the floor, pulling the base of your spine out of your pelvis.
4 Pull in your tummy muscles tight, rounding your low back, and attempt to stretch your coccyx towards the floor, from the base of your spine down. Movement here will be incremental but significant.
5 Hold for 60 seconds, breathing softly.

Legs passing

If your back is painful, this exercise will help your hips swing freely and make walking easier. It also encourages the abdominal muscles to hold the pillar of lumbar segments secure as the legs move, protecting the low back from ongoing micro-trauma during everyday life. The exercise is an effective way of tricking the tummy muscles to switch on when they resist because of back pain. It is a very important first exercise for getting the tummy muscles working again. Make a mental note of the degree to which they are working and attempt to replicate this when you are up and walking about. This is how your tummy should work!

1 Lie on your back on a soft carpeted floor, bringing your arms up and crossing them behind your head.
2 Tighten your tummy muscles and press your low back into the floor as you bring your left knee towards your left armpit with the knee fully bent.

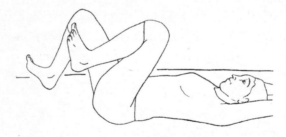

3 As your return the left leg to the floor, lift the right leg so the legs pass mid-air. Do not let your returning foot rest on the floor between excursions and do not straighten either knee at any stage as this strains your low back. You will feel the midriff fully switched on as you control the weighty legs passing one another.
4 Continue for 60 seconds, moving the legs slowly and with control.

Intermediate

Segmental pelvic bridging

This exercise restores the pliability of your spine, helping it work segmentally rather than as a rod cast rigid by pain. It literally breaks the hold of muscle spasm and allows the segments to start jostling beside one another and pulling apart. It is very effective for restoring segmental control when the small intrinsic muscles have atrophied due to the spine moving as a block. Segmental movement also induces pressure changes through the discs and keeps them healthy. As the spinal segments draw away and compress like a concertina, the discs suck and squirt fluid, which improves their nutrition. Your low back often feels tight after a few repetitions of this exercise, so you should always follow with the 'Knees rocking' exercise (on page 45) and 'Reverse curl-ups' (on page 50).

1 Lie on your back on a soft carpeted floor with your knees bent and your feet placed as close as possible to your bottom. Your arms should be over your head with the fingers interlaced and your palms turned away.

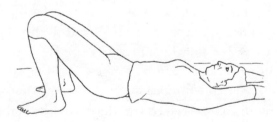

2 Clench your buttocks and pull in your tummy muscles tight as you tip your pelvis back, making your low back into a round wheel.
3 Pressing your low back into the floor, roll up your spine, one cog at a time. Try to feel each segment in turn meeting the floor, particularly the recessed ones which won't press easily into the carpet.
4 Continue rolling right up your spine to the base of your neck one

cog at a time, until your body forms a straight line between shoulders, hips and knees. Rest comfortably, taking weight on the prominent bump at the base of your neck.

5   Remain in this position for 15 seconds. It is important to keep

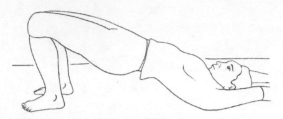

your gluteal muscles switched on by pinning your knees together.

6   Initiate the return journey by making a horizontal crease across your belly at navel level by sucking your tummy in hard.

7   Fold your back down to the floor, one cog at a time, distinctly feeling your spine pass over each spinal segment. It is always difficult to press the back at waist-level into the floor.

8   Repeat roll up and down twice.

Reverse curl-ups

Reverse curl-ups strengthen the lower abdominals instead of the oft-used upper abdominals (as done in normal sit-ups and crunches). Overworking the upper abdominals causes the upper body to stoop over and leaves a pouchy underbelly below the navel; in other words it accentuates poor posture. Reverse curl-ups strengthen the oblique abdominals and transversus abdominus (the intermediate and deep abdominal muscle layers), which exert a more direct control on the spinal segments. As they strengthen, they shrink the abdomen at the front—helping to create a thinner hour-glass waist—as they allow opening of the spinal interspaces at the back, thus performing two important actions in one.

1   Lie on your back on the floor, pulling your thighs up to your chest with your ankles crossed and your knees apart. Interlace your fingers behind your head.

2   Without jerking, lift your bottom off the floor and your knees

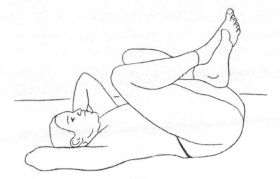

towards your chin and then return your thighs to the start position. Do not let your thighs go beyond vertical to the floor on the way down as this will strain your lower back.

3   Repeat 15 times, bringing your legs up and down at the same speed, though you will find it much harder to lower the legs slowly. If you have a neck problem you will need to prevent strain travelling upwards by putting your hands, palms upwards, on your forehead instead of behind your neck.

The BackBlock

This is the classic posture to counteract the strains of sitting in the same position for hours. It is most effective at the end of the day or after any long period (greater than 2 hours) of sitting, when the discs have suffered great fluid loss. It is a spinal decompressing exercise and it primarily opens the front of the spinal interspaces and effects marked pressure changes through the lumbar discs. In the long-term this stimulates disc metabolism, principally the synthesis of proteoglycans, which bolsters disc hydration and ultimately disc nutrition. In the short term, it sucks water into the lumbar discs and delays the desiccation and disc flattening that occurs through the course of each day. It is also important to do this exercise to decompress your spine after running or standing about for long periods. *See* page 239 for where to buy a BackBlock.

1   Lie on the floor on your back with your knees bent.

2 Lift your bottom off the floor by rolling up the spine, one cog at a time, until your body forms a straight line between shoulders, hips and knees (*see* 'Segmental pelvic bridging' above).

3 Slide the BackBlock under your bottom and roll down the spine, coming gently to rest on the block on your way down. Make sure you don't position the BackBlock too high up your spine: it should *not* rest under the vertebrae themselves but under the sacrum, that hard flat bone at the bottom of your spine.

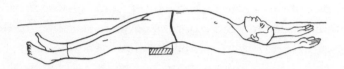

4 Gradually straighten each leg out along the floor by pushing your heel away from the block. Do not lift your legs as you straighten them as this strains the low back.

5 Completely let go when you are in position over the BackBlock; the greater the relaxation the greater the segmental separation. Depending on your degree of kink, both the front of your hips and your low back, you will feel a pulling sensation in your low back, almost as though your legs are pulling the pelvis off the base of your spine. You should feel an agreeable discomfort, though it may sometimes be difficult to stay in position for more than a few seconds if the pulling is great. It should not be agony but it should feel as though it means business; as if it goes straight to the nub of things.

6 After 60 seconds, or less if you cannot tolerate it, bend your knees slowly, one at a time, and lift up your bottom as you slide the Back-Block away. Lower your bottom to the floor, one cog at a time, just as you did when lifting up. It always hurts to raise your bottom off the BackBlock. Don't be fazed by this: the longer you have been lying there the more it will hurt to lift off.

7 Do the 'Knees rocking' exercise (page 45) for 30 seconds and 15 'Reverse curl-ups' (page 50) after coming off the BackBlock.

If you fail to do these exercises afterwards you will be sore!
8 Repeat twice.

Squatting

Squatting pulls the spinal interspaces apart without invoking the muscle hold of 'Curl-downs' (*see* following exercise), which to a degree compresses the spinal segments. Squatting creates pressure changes through the lumbar discs that stimulate metabolic activity. It is a quick way to decompress the spine through the day; thwarting the slow settling of the segments as the discs gradually lose fluid. Squatting is the evolutionary precursor to sitting and the spine's natural way of pulling itself apart after it has been compressed by upright postures.

1 With your feet parallel and big toes together, drop your bottom to the floor, holding a secure surface or rail as you do to keep you steady.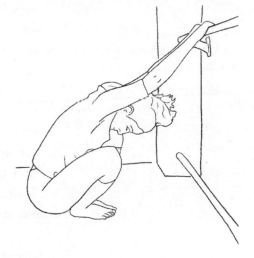
2 Part your knees wide, letting your head drop through towards the floor.
3 Suck your tummy in like a greyhound and make small bouncing movements, attempting to get your bottom closer to the floor.
4 Continue for 15 to 30 seconds, trying to elongate your spine with each downward movement.
5 Return to the standing position by reefing in the tummy muscles hard and pushing up through your thighs. The knees will complain initially but within a few days of doing this exercise they will love it (the pressure changes are good for them too!).
6 Repeat twice.

Advanced

Curl-downs and unfurling to vertical
(also known as 'Toe touches')

This important exercise reintroduces the spine to controlled bending. It pulls the spinal segments apart, giving the discs a drink, and re-educates the power of the small spinal intrinsic muscles (particularly multifidus). These span the spinal interspaces and keep the segments stable, so they don't painfully shear forwards as the spine bends. Important and essential as intrinsic control is, rehabilitation can make the back ache more for a few days, which is often misinterpreted as being bad for the back and makes people shy away from doing what is necessary. Once you have done this exercise, always follow with the 'Knees rocking' and 'Rolling along your spine' exercises (pages 46–7) to disperse the soreness.

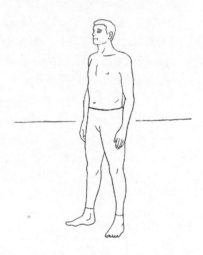

1 Standing upright, brace your tummy to reduce the tendency for segmental forward shear (the strength gained through your reverse curl-ups will help you here) and curl your body down towards your toes. Tighten your buttocks as you go forwards. If you feel too weak to do it comfortably you can walk your hands down your thighs until you can hang more easily.

2 Round your low back to make a horizontal crease across your belly at navel level. Bend low enough to hang. This is where your spinal control passes from the spinal muscles to the ligaments and you get maximal vertebral separation.

3 Bend your knees for greater comfort, dangling like a gorilla. Be sure to completely relax, letting your spine pull out so you hang on your straps.

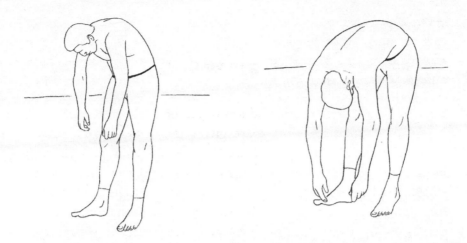

4 Let the spine lengthen as you relax and bounce very gently for 5 seconds.
5 Pull the tummy in hard, tightening the gluteal muscles, and start to unfurl. Hump your low back as you unwind and keep your chin on the chest to the very last. Take care to resist the temptation to arch back and flip yourself up through the last few degrees of straightening. Keep the movement under slow control, with your midriff strong and tightened all the way.
6 Repeat twice only, morning and afternoon, particularly when your back feels it is starting to get tight. Although this exercise restores essential lost function, too many repetitions will make you sore. Progress is a delicate balance and you must listen to your instincts.

The floor twists

This exercise helps realign spinal segments that have become fixed in a small degree of axial rotation. Holding your foot in your hand encourages the tails of the lumbar vertebrae to swing to the other side of midline. This normalises faulty spinal function and helps deal with pain. Floor twists also open out the facet joints along the upper side of the spine, which can become inflamed as a result of the twisted sit of their vertebrae. At the same time straightening the upper leg at the knee exerts traction of the lumbar nerve roots and pulls them free of their exit canal. This helps combat nerve root tethering, which often goes with facet joint arthropathy (the nerve sheath adheres to the inflamed facet capsule). Where axial rotation is blocked to one side, you must repeat the stretch to that side four times more than the freer side to restore balance.

1 Lie on your back on a soft-carpeted floor with your arms outstretched from the shoulders at right angles, palms facing down. Make sure you have a lot of space around you to do the exercise.
2 Bring both knees onto your chest, one at a time, and then take them over to your right side so that they rest on the floor, keeping your knees high up to your body, as close to your chin as possible, and together. Your thighs should be parallel on the floor while you straighten your uppermost (left) leg at the knee.

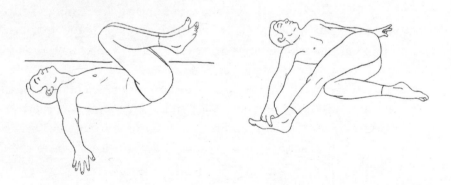

3 Attempt to hold the toes of your foot with your right hand. If you cannot reach the toes, hold behind your calf or knee, rather than bending the knee to reach your toes. Try to keep the palm of your left hand flat down on the carpet which (often painfully) opens the front of this shoulder as the pectoral area stretches.
4 When in position, make small adjustments to get your upper back twisted back flatter, in closer contact with the floor.
5 Remain in position for 30 seconds, attempting to breathe into the base of your lungs, then return to step 2.
6 Repeat to the other side and once again to each side.

Child's pose to cobra

This exercise rightly belongs in the advanced category. When you first attempt to get your bottom to your heels you will find that your back has difficulty letting go. The long spinal muscles at the spine's base are slow to switch off and it can be painful accommodating the extreme postural change. This is all very normal; you will find your lower back adjusts more readily as its function starts to improve. Simply take it slowly and wait for things to relax as your bottom sits down on your heels.

1 From the position of the 'Child's pose' exercise (page 47) slide your outstretched arms back so that your hands are underneath your shoulders on the floor.

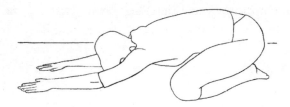

2 Pull your tummy in tight and hump your lower back, lifting your bottom off your heels.

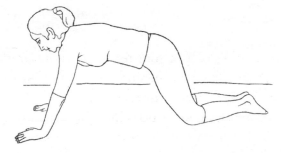

3 Take your weight forward on your arms and let your groin fall through towards the floor. Do not let your elbows bend as your arms take weight and deliberately make your gluteal muscles relax as you let go of your low back.

4 Try to let your low back 'hang through' in a deep hollow, with all the muscles relaxed. This may take a while, as your back lets go in stages, almost in jerks as it passes through the more rigid, middle phase.

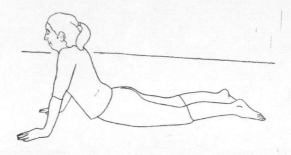

5 Remain in the hanging position for 30 seconds, feeling the spine silently settling into a hollow.
6 Revert to the original 'Child's pose' position by pulling the tummy in hard to protect your spine and pushing your weight back towards your heels as you pass through the kneeling position.
7 Attempt to push your sitting bones through the seat of your pants as you elongate your spine back until your bottom is comfortably nestling on your heels.

Chapter two
Your thoracic spine

WHAT IS YOUR THORACIC SPINE?

Your thoracic spine is the middle part of your back. It starts from just below C7, the prominent bump at the base of the neck, and extends down to waist level where your lumbar spine begins. The thoracic spine gives you the most visible 'look' of your posture, the ramrod straight back of the sergeant major, the round-shouldered hunch of the slouch, or the many stances in between.

The role of the thoracic spine is twofold: first it supports the chest cage, which expands and contracts with breathing, and, second, it provides a mobile base for the neck so it can carry the unwieldy head without strain. Both these roles face difficulty if alignment of the thoracic spine is below par.

Spinal alignment and good posture play a critical role in spinal function—poor alignment and posture conversely play a role in the genesis of pain. Side on, the spine should exhibit a gentle S bend from top to bottom, with a scoop for the neck (cervical lordosis), a rounded chest curve (thoracic kyphosis) and a hollow in the low back (lumbar lordosis). Former generations have led us to believe that upright posture and a straight back was somehow 'better for you' but from a biomechanical view this is not the case. For the thorax—and the spine above and below—to work optimally your thoracic spine should have a gently rounded hump from the base of the neck to the waist, with the rib cage gently hanging off either side.

Your twelve thoracic vertebrae are smaller and more delicate than your lumbar brethren, and their side projections (transverse processes) are also longer and finer. Their backward projecting tails (spinous processes) slope downwards, overlapping one another like thatches of a roof, instead of pointing back horizontally, as they do in the neck and the lumbar region. The overlap of thoracic spinous processes restricts your range of backward arching (extension).

Twelve ribs are attached to either side of your thoracic vertebrae, actually straddling the intervertebral disc. This rib-joining arrangement is noteworthy because it impedes spinal mobility, especially bending forward (flexion) and side bending. To add further clutter in tethering your chest cage to the spine, your ribs also make glancing connection with the tips of the lateral struts projecting out either side of your vertebrae (transverse processes), as they circle the chest to meet your breastbone (sternum) at the front.

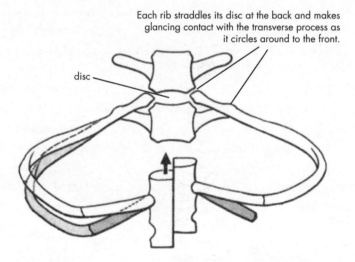

FIGURE 2.1 The ribs are like bucket handles which move up and out as we breathe in, and down and in as we breathe out.

Your first ribs start high up the spine, at about the level a necklace is worn at the base of the neck (people are always surprised they begin so high). The first ribs are like small crooked fingers and you can feel them by digging into the web of muscle in your neck-shoulder junction. All your ribs pass down and forwards as they curve around the side of your chest wall, before becoming cartilaginous at the front to meld in with the sternum.

The ribs make your chest into a semi-collapsible cage, just like a chicken carcass, and your chest volume is increased and decreased by muscle action. A breath 'in' is brought about by your dome-shaped diaphragm contracting and descending into your abdomen. The increased chest capacity reduces the pressure within the pleural space, so air flows in and the lungs inflate. After a breathable amount of air has passed in, you pause and then exhale; the 'out' breath happening when your muscles relax. The elastic recoil of your diaphragm and rib cage lets your lungs return to their resting volume, thereby expelling a quantity of stale air.

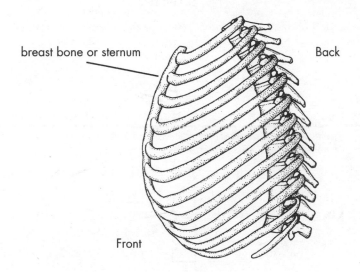

breast bone or sternum

Back

Front

FIGURE 2.2 Side view of thoracic spine showing the expandable rib cage.

You can see, therefore, that lung capacity and efficiency of breathing are directly related to the freedom of the chest hinges (joints) and elasticity of the soft tissues. This is just as important to our mental processes—and sense of wellbeing—as it is to the more tangibly important issues, like getting oxygen in for the body's metabolism and expelling the waste gases (mostly carbon dioxide).

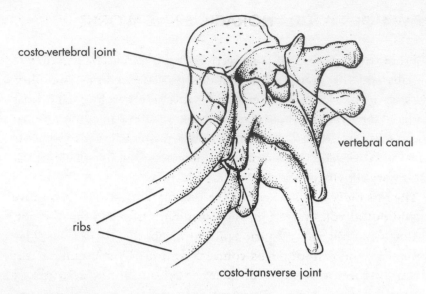

costo-vertebral joint

vertebral canal

ribs

costo-transverse joint

FIGURE 2.3 **The sweep of the ribs makes joints at the vertebral body (costo-vertebral joint) and the transverse processes (costo-transverse joint).**

Your autonomic nervous system is a lacework of nerves that drapes over the rib-to-spine (costo-vertebral) junctions on both sides. The less-discernable function of your visceral organs is governed by this system. Thoracic (mechanical) disorder can affect both your internal functions—such as digestion—and the autonomic function of your arms, such as dilation of blood, sweating and goose flesh. Unimportant as these functions may seem, cumulative effects of their disturbed function can adversely influence your arms' soft tissue vitality.

Poor thoracic function reduces the viability at the hard-working 'hot spots' of the arms, which then manifest as various soft-tissue disorders. There may be low-grade pain and stiffness in the mid-back, extending over many years, which seemed to bear no relation to complaints of tennis elbow, say, or carpal tunnel syndrome, Dupytren's contracture (tightening of the palm) and various tendon sheath problems. The 'lead arms' syndrome of kayakers, who sit bolt upright using powerful scapula work to paddle, is in the same order of complaint. Treatment must address the poor function of the thoracic spine first, rather than working on the effects, to be successful.

HOW DOES YOUR THORACIC SPINE WORK?

The thoracic is the least mobile section of the spine. The presence of the ribs and the shape of the spinous processes hamper mobility, particularly of flexion and extension and side bending. The least hindered movement is twist (axial rotation) because here the ribs can spread away from one another in a transverse plane as the segments swivel on their axes. All thoracic movement incorporates continual respiratory activity of the ribs.

The ribs move like bucket handles during respiration. They move up and out as you breathe in, and down and in as you breathe out, so that whatever the thoracic spine does in the way of everyday movement, the respiring ribs come along too. This is quite a feat of coordination, when you consider the life-sustaining activities of the chest cage. It carries on relentlessly sucking in fresh air and expelling stale, while at the same time both ribs and thoracic spine must accommodate all sorts of other less essential tasks—be it shrugging your shoulders to music, cleaning the windows, or throwing a javelin.

Apart from its role in supporting the chest cage and accommodating respiratory and other elective chest activity, the thoracic spine provides background mobility for the free-swinging head. Although the neck itself is fantastically mobile, it relies heavily on the mobile-base properties of the thorax. By being positioned under the neck and going some way towards overall movement, the thoracic spine sets the stage for the much more flamboyant movement above.

As described in the previous chapter, generosity of movement is made possible higher up through the spine by the centre of movement of each vertebra locating slightly further forward of its neighbour below. This means the spinal column possesses phenomenal bending-over mobility at the top, and some people can even bring their nose to their knees! The same applies on a smaller scale with the neck on the thorax, and without this deep-seated input from the thoracic spine, our necks would have a fraction of their range. They would suffer insupportable wear and tear where the heavy block of the cranium sits on the neck and also where the neck joins the less compliant and boxy thorax.

WHAT ARE THE ACCESSORY MOVEMENTS OF YOUR THORACIC SPINE?

All accessory movements of the vertebrae are important in the thoracic spine, because it is a relatively tight barrel. All twelve vertebrae and their pairs of ribs must have their full quota of mobility, otherwise the cloying constriction of this complex festoonery of attachments further reduces available freedom.

The most valuable accessory movement of your thorax is swivel, or axial twist. Thoracic vertebrae glide and tip as they do in other parts of the spine, though less generously. Twisting is the freest movement and it harbours the greatest potential to drag your ribs along too. Thus, twisting exercises the ribs most; keeping their joints patent and the lungs able to expand. It is important to bear in mind that providing mobility to suck and release the gases involved in your body's metabolic processes is your chest's chief physical role.

Your ribs are lashed on to the sides of the spine by a criss-cross tethering of ligaments. And though it is important for the ribs to hold on, they quickly cause problems if they hold on too tight. A stiff costo-vertebral junction can be an ample source of pain. It also creates a drier, stiffer disc and causes a stiff spinal segment as the buoyancy of the disc diminishes and the vertebra sitting on top becomes sluggish. As you saw in the previous chapter, hypomobility of a segment leads to poor nutrition, which leads to disc degeneration, which in turn escalates pain.

A single rib commonly loses mobility as the result of a one-off wrenching incident. Intense muscle exertion can pull a rib slightly askew at one or all of its several points of attachment to the spine and leave the costo-vertebral junction stiff. Thereafter your rib becomes less compliant and stubbornly painful, like a dagger between the ribs. From my experience, a nagging pain like this accounts for the wide variety of pains in all different parts of the chest wall that are commonly misdiagnosed. I have seen gall bladders removed in search of the source of such a pain.

Practised therapists can always feel a stiffer rib. It sits up proud from the others, like a cable around a barrel, and it is harder to manually depress. The attached vertebra is usually more recessed and feels like a piano key that won't come up. It is often stuck in axial rotation, with its tail left or right of centre. Transverse pressures from the deviated side will feel free, like a door swinging through, but locked and bolted from the other way. Pressure on the free direction side will be painless but uncomfortable and loath to go from the other.

The thoracic area is easier to palpate accurately than the other parts of your spine, simply because everything is so near the surface. The vertebrae are more prominent and their spinous processes obvious as a familiar row of knobs through the skin. It is possible for someone to do a cursory sweep down your back, tapping each knob in turn with the fingers to tell which is stiffer, like sounding with a tuning fork. It is possible to tell the degree of stiffness by the sound each segment makes, almost like the different frequencies of each musical note. The problem area often exerts a drag on the fingers as they are swept down the spine in one full movement. This probably indicates a patch of skin that is more damp, caused by a low-grade inflammation lying underneath.

If the rib is stiff, the corresponding vertebra and costo-vertebral joint will be implicated. The costo-vertebral joints exist beside the spine, between each spinous process, about 1 centimetre out. In its problem state, it feels thicker and more hardened to probing thumb pressures, whereas the joint of the healthy side feels empty and painless.

The superficial boniness of the thoracic area makes releasing a gummed up costo-vertebral junction unusually painful. Effective mobilising is better achieved from afar, using a longer lever by working at the rib angle, where the rib abruptly changes direction nearer the sidewall of the chest. Because of the complex bowing and contorting line of the rib, downward thumb pressures at the rib angle causes complex movement at the costo-vertebral hinge. Rib angle treatment pressures are very effective at releasing ribs from the spine.

HOW DOES THE THORACIC SPINE GO WRONG?

Anomalies of spinal curvature are a fundamental cause of pain in the thoracic area. Thoracic spines that are too flat or too hunched cause pain, as does spinal scoliosis, with its lateral to and fro twisting bends (when viewed from behind). A too-flat thoracic spine causes less pain than a kyphotic or scoliotic one but the ill-effects for the neck may be greater (*see* next chapter). The distribution of pain from a kyphosis is more predictable than a scoliotic spine, which varies greatly with the complexity of the curve.

With an over-kyphotic thoracic spine the spine humps out at the back and the shoulders draw forward. The condition often goes with the stoop associated with extreme tallness, though over-active accessory muscles of respiration can also be a cause, which is seen in chronic pulmonary conditions such as asthma, emphysema or bronchitis. The hunch of the upper back often goes with an over-inflated chest cage, caused by air-hunger, and the hitching up of the shoulders, which also shortens the neck. Once the posture causes the head to project forward, in front of the line of gravity, the stoop can accelerate rapidly due to the weight of the upper body bearing down. As you will read in the next chapter, this posture also causes neck problems through over-activity of the upper trapezius (muscle) trying to control the head.

The spinous processes flare apart at the back around the hump, like fish scales opening out, and the chest is stiffly resistant to arching backwards (extension). The widening of the gap at the back of the interspaces causes the facet surfaces to slide apart and chronically stretches the costo-vertebral junction where it straddles a disc. This causes the rib joints to stiffen as does the increased hoop tension of the long paraspinal muscles as they stretch around the hump of the kyphosis.

All the vertebrae are stiff with an over-kyphotic thoracic spine but the apical segment is always the most extreme. The discs near the apex of the curve may develop wedge deformity as their metabolism is retarded as a result of the unremitting pressures. Eventually, the vertebral bodies develop wedging as well, since bone is like dense plastic and modifies its shape according the pressures exerted upon it. These principles should also be borne in mind during rehabilitation, when using the BackBlock to stretch the spine straighter.

Wedging of the vertebral bodies is often associated with irregularities of the vertebral end-plate (the flat cartilaginous interface between disc and vertebra). Evidence on scans of tear-drop depressions in the vertebral body extending up from the end-plate (Schmorl's nodes) indicates a previous minute breach of the plate and rupture into the honeycomb bone of the body. This may make the vertebral end-plate irregular and furry on X-rays. It also makes it less permeable to diffusion of nutrients from the reservoirs in the vertebral bodies. This speeds degeneration of the discs.

With a too-straight thoracic spine the ribs fail to approach from the optimum angle for their anatomical alignment and the junction they make is a difficult one. As the ribs' movement becomes more laboured, the costo-vertebral strain manifests as pain in different patches over the back of the chest wall. Stiffness may be heightened if the straightness of the mid-back causes the spinous processes to lie down overlapping one another, almost touching. Although the 'kissing spines' do not cause pain they impede mobility and bunch together the costo-vertebral joints. The too-straight back also puts the scapula-to-spine muscles into a shortened position, making it harder to get effective strength from the arms. The area between the shoulder blades can look over-muscled, with a dark-shadowed groove down the mid-line.

A too-straight thoracic spine also fails to provide optimal background posture for the neck and makes it harder for the neck to assume a lordotic arch. As you will read in the next chapter, this causes the neck to jar because it cannot sink and spring during upright activity to ride out impact.

With a scoliotic thoracic spine, the spine develops lateral twisting S-shaped curvature, which may be congenital or acquired through a difference in leg length. The bucking spine pinches the sides of the vertebrae in its lateral hoops. It also causes the vertebrae to twist on their axes—one way below the apex, the other above.

A thoracic scoliosis is often secondary—and concave in the opposite direction—to a primary curvature below in the lumbar spine. Thus, the spine exhibits two lateral hoops, concave in opposite directions—each curve holding a vertebra tightly pinched at its apex. The apical segment is always the stiffest and is often recessed. It may be exquisitely tender and so locked away it is difficult to get at with thumbs. The pain of the apical segment is usually central, though the twisted vertebrae above and below can refer pain laterally, and lower than the problem spinal level. In this instance patients are often surprised that the culprit vertebra is so much higher in the back than where their pain manifests to the side.

With a scoliotic spine the ribs encounter great difficulty keying into the twisting and buckling sides, because the vertebrae are both side-tilted and rotated on their axes. It is not possible to be pedantic about where the pain will spray, though the most painful ribs are usually prominent.

With treatment for scoliosis, all the ribs and stiff spinal segments need systematic loosening with manual mobilisation, as an adjunct to spinal stretching regimes. Mobilising pressures are effective both at the rib angle and directly on the costo-vertebral junctions. When the body senses irritability of a rib, it invokes protective muscle spasm of the local intercostals (the muscles between the ribs). The tonic hold of the muscles oozes the rib outwards to make it more prominent, like one rung of a ladder sitting proud of the others. This is uncomfortable and feels like a tight band around the chest.

The spasm immediately lessens the rib excursions and makes breathing shallower. Just one stiff rib can cause the entire chest cage to become less elastic, making it easy to see, incidentally, why it is so important to get the posture of asthmatic children right. It is also possible that chronic rib stiffness can be the cause of the recurrent collapse of specific lobes of the lung that goes with chronic chest conditions with large volumes of secretions (bronchiectasis and pneumonia). It is important to point out that over-energetic coughing can also strain ribs, thereafter leaving them less compliant at their costo-vertebral junction, and thus putting the patient into double jeopardy from both pain and infection.

Poor functioning of the costo-vertebral joints causes a variety of aches and pains in a rainbow distribution down the mid-back, depending on which spinal level is at fault. A stiff rib can elude detection for years and may be the source of a stubborn, nagging pain, which a spouse is often recruited to rub or massage. It is always more noticeable when the back is tired and typically feels like a stitch as the cordy muscles around it keep it pushed up and sore.

As the problem gets worse, pain may spread around the side of the chest wall between the ribs in a girdle distribution. Or, it can pierce right through to the front of the chest and surface through the sternum like a knife. Both pains can be brought on by a deep breath and it is tempting to take shallow breaths to avoid provoking it. Nagging as the problem is, it responds quickly to mobilising pressures.

With thoracic scoliosis and kyphosis it is also possible to feel pain at the front of the chest at the costo-chondral junctions, where the ribs join the sternum. This can also be caused by excessive sleeping on one side, where the weight of the body causes bunching of one side of the chest on the mattress. Once again, the stiff rib will sit higher than the others at the front of the chest and resist manual pressures.

THE COMMON DISORDERS OF THE THORACIC SPINE

Stiff spinal segments of a thoracic kyphosis

Increase in the rounding of the back in the thoracic area is usually associated with drooping shoulders and the head carried too far forward, in front of the line of gravity. This can be an inherited congenital condition or acquired later in life by lazy habits of posture. In addition to the pain of a trapped apical vertebra, the postural strain of this condition creates a pain at the base of the neck and across the top of the shoulders. This pain is caused by overwork of the muscles in holding the head back when the angle in the spine at the top of the back directs the line of vision to the floor.

The trapezeii muscles, which run from the base of the skull down either side of the neck to fan out across the shoulders, have the job of bracing the shoulder blades and keeping the head back, retracted in line with the shoulders. With advanced thoracic kyphosis, trapezius bilaterally is forced to act like horse's reins to pull the head back over the support of the spine below. But because the head is so heavy and because so many activities, especially precision ones, involve bowing the head forward over a small field of vision, this is a tall order.

The constant postural strain makes muscles develop a low-grade tension, which keeps the underlying vertebrae permanently bunched together. Over time, the intervertebral discs compress and become drier as they lose fluid. A dull gnawing pain develops at the cross-bar of the shoulders from several spinal segments stiffening, like cotton reels stuck together. There can also be a different pain, like a hot twinge, from the cramp of the muscles clenching. This pain is from muscle fatigue as distinct from a joint pain, which makes you want to arch your head back for relief.

A similar pain can develop across the base of the neck when using the arms unsupported but the reasons for this are slightly different. This problem is mostly encountered by people who work for long periods holding their arms up. Pianists and computer operators spend hours with their arms poised aloft over a keyboard. Pain is usually located at the base of the neck, on the side of the dominant hand. It can be heightened by anxiety and tension and also by heavy carrying, such as shopping.

Rib dysfunction with a sergeant major's back

Too-straight thoracic spines tend to develop difficulties with the ribs keying into the spine, rather than jamming of the spinal segments. Because of the close proximity of the spinous processes, which almost touch as they lie down over one another like fish scales, an over-straight thoracic spine tends to jack open the segmental interspaces. While opening the front of the disc spaces, this alignment also tends to 'crowd the back', which includes the difficult union made with the ribs.

One of the far-reaching effects of this is disturbance of the auto-nomic function of the arms. The autonomic nervous system regulates automatic activity such as the diameter of blood vessels and the phenomena of sweating and goose flesh. The nervous lacework of this system drapes itself in a chain down either side of the spine, just superficial to (nearer the surface) the costo-vertebral junctions.

It is thought that poor functional performance of these junctions causes disturbed function of the autonomic nervous system, which can bring about a variety of symptoms in the arms. The best descrip-tion of these symptoms is simply that the arms 'don't feel part of you'. The arms can feel heavy 'like lead' and you lack the strength to keep them up to work. But you can also experience numbness and pain, typically in a glove distribution through the forearms and hands. This is often associated with feelings of the hands being cold, or the veins standing up on the back of the hands. You can also get similar symptoms with markedly rounded upper back, though this postural anomaly has to be quite severe.

Heavy breastedness is often a feature in the syndrome of a too-straight thoracic spine. A large and heavy bosom creates a bowing or crumpling forward of the upper back, with the result that the spinal muscles have to work overtime to keep the spine straight. This compensatory effect can make the thoracic spine too straight, which then crowds the spinal segments at the back, making the costovertebral junctions stiff. In addition, the bra straps on the shoulders can add to the compression of the thoracic column, which becomes an additional cause of segmental jamming.

Segmental stiffness and rib dysfunction of spinal scoliosis

Spinal scoliosis can be responsible for diffuse pain, both locally at the front and back of the thorax, and far reaching, in the form of headaches and leg pain (sciatica). The cause lies in the factors outlined above: disturbances of spinal alignment. The lateral deviations of the spine cause both segmental stiffness and inflammation where the ribs slot into the spine.

Scoliosis has the appearance of a frozen wave of movement through the spine. There is a static twisting and buckling of the column throughout its length. The lack of equilibrium makes the stacked vertebrae slew around insidiously on one another, pinching together at the front and sides. Drastic as it may sound, scoliosis need not be severe. Mild scoliosis is extremely common; so much so that radiologists often fail to comment on their presence in X-ray reports. However, I believe even mild scoliosis can be a prolific source of pain.

There are several parts of a scoliotic spine that cause trouble. Firstly, the vertebrae at the apex of each lateral curve pinch together on the inside concavity of the curve where disc nutrition is impaired and metabolism slows. Above and below the apex there is a sideways shearing strain in the leaning sections of spine, as they slip one way below the apex and the opposite way above. In addition there is a twisting moment to each vertebra, which bends laterally. As a vertebra tilts sideways to the left, say, its tail moves across-ways to the right. So another source of pain occurs at the levels of the spine with the greatest fixed twist of a vertebra. And as we already know, more pain comes from the rib junctions, as the working ribs attempt to key themselves into the sides of a bucking and rolling spine.

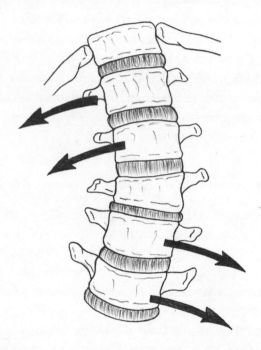

FIGURE 2.4 Spinal scoliosis pinches the apical vertebra and the segments slide laterally one way below the apex and the other way above.

The pain is a conglomeration of those described in kyphotic and too-straight spines but the distribution is more extensive. In fact the feature of scoliotic spines is pain everywhere. Children are often dismissed as malingerers when they describe a pain that criss-crosses left and right from the skull down to the base of the spine, with headaches and sciatic pains in the legs also. However, this litany of symptoms is usually sadly accurate.

WHAT CAN YOU DO ABOUT IT?

In rectifying these common problems of the upper back we must correct the abnormalities of spinal alignment. This is easier said than done, of course. All the conditions described above have been acquired over time and it is not a simple matter to undo them by the wave of a wand. However, the good news is that even the slightest degree of loosening of the tight structures will start to bring relief. Quite quickly, you will sense a greater freedom of movement and the pain fading. Even if pain is not an issue for you and you simply do not like the look of your back or the way you stand, the same exercises will bring benefits. If the back is too rounded, you must get it to go straighter. If the back is too straight, you must introduce some bend, and if it is twisted, you must work towards prising it out straight.

Beginners

The right angle

This exercise helps align the spine and is especially effective for a round-shouldered back with tight pectoral muscles at the front of the chest that pull your shoulders forward. It is also effective at pulling the lumbar nerve roots clear of their exit canals. It may be difficult to keep your bottom on the floor if you have tight hamstrings. As a semi-inverted yoga pose that rests the legs and drains stale blood from your ankles, it is a nice way to relax before starting a complete exercise regime.

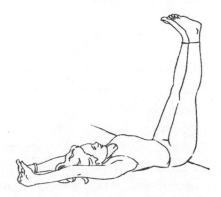

1 Find a clear space of wall with some uncluttered floor in front of it. Sit sideways into the wall with your bottom as close to it as possible.
2 Roll onto your back and swing your legs up the wall,

stretching your arms out along the floor above your head. You should find yourself in a right-angled bend at the hips. Do not allow your knees to bend or your bottom to lift off the floor.

3   Hold this position for 2 to 5 minutes. You can make this exercise more taxing by interlacing your fingers and turning the hands away, above your head—keeping the arms parallel and not bending your elbows. You can also go one further by doing the 'Angel's wings stretch' (page 81–2) while in position by taking your arms down to your hips in a wide semi-circle, the backs of your hands in contact with the carpet all the way around. Try to breathe out as they go down and in as they come up.

4   To release, bend your legs on the wall, and round your back. With your knees bent, tip onto your side on the floor. Note that the longer you have been in this position, the more fixed you will feel on release. Make small wriggling movements on your side to soften your spine before getting up.

Rolling up the wall

This exercise follows on from the previous one and is the exercise of choice if you are not fit enough to get into 'The plough' pose (page 79–80). It mobilises the thoracic segments one by one, like fingers rolling over a keyboard, and helps make the chest cage more compliant. As you guide yourself up your spine you will learn to tarry over flat patches and where vertebrae are painfully prominent or recessed. As you roll over the ribs, you may feel one side is more rigid than the other. This is an indication to roll up and down more on this side. This exercise also strengthens the small intrinsic muscles of the spine, as well as the gluteal muscles of your buttocks, making it easier to achieve core stability.

1   From the previous position of your feet up the wall, bend one leg then the other, to make an obtuse angle at both knees, feet flat on the wall.

2   With arms straight above your head, fingers interlaced and palms turned away, pull your shoulder blades around to the side of your chest wall so that you don't roll on them.

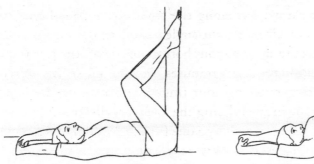
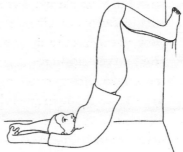

3   Pull your tummy in tight and tip your pelvis back to round your low back and roll up your spine.

4   Try to get right up your spine to C7, the prominent bump at the base of your neck, making your body form a straight line between your shoulders, hips and knees. Do not hunch your shoulders; try to get the sense of bearing weight through your shoulders and upper ribs. This will cause a marked stretching sensation at the back of your neck.

5   Hold this position for 30 seconds, keeping your buttocks clenched to push your pelvis forward, and then roll down your spine, one cog at a time, to rest your bottom on the floor.

6   Repeat twice. Note: Do *not* move your head while doing this exercise.

The floor-sitting twist

This exercise helps disengage the ribs from the sides of the thoracic segments. You often sense one rib in particular will not let go, and it may be easier to twist one way than the other.

1   Sit on the floor with both legs stretched out straight in front

2   Bending your right knee, place your right foot on the floor to the outside of your left knee, your left hand on the floor behind you.

3   Drag your navel across to the left and, pushing your

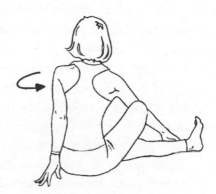

right elbow on the inside of your right knee, twist your upper body to the left.

4 Go as far as you can, then pull your tummy in and go one more notch to the left.

5 Hold for 30 seconds.

6 Repeat in the opposite direction. then repeat twice in both directions.

7 At full twist, include a transverse side glide through the length of your chest cage. This is an incremental side-bowing action, first one way then the other, which glides the spinal segments left and right and helps free the stiffer rib. You often feel a shriller pain when you include this movement.

The tennis ball release

A faulty rib junction behaves exactly like a rusty hinge, so it will respond beautifully if you apply direct pressure to the hinge itself. You will need a new tennis ball for this exercise.

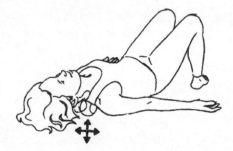

1 Lie on your back on the floor with your knees bent and feet flat on the ground.

2 Rise up slightly to manoeuvre the ball under yourself, so it sits exactly under the painful spot, near the spine.

3 Lower some of your weight down onto the ball and wriggle around on it so that it agitates the rusty rib function as you roll back and forth over it. Make the movements of the ball small so that you spend most of the time with the ball exactly under that painful spot. There will be a sweet pain: agony but ecstasy.

4 Continue for as long as you can bear it but for no more than 3 minutes to avoid bruising.

Intermediate

The thoracic arms tangle

This exercise helps release tight muscles across the top of your shoulders but is most effective in dragging the ribs laterally off the spine in the mid to lower thoracic area. It is helpful for scoliotic spines as well as a too-straight back.

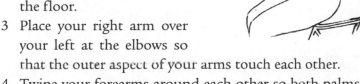

1 Sit towards the front of a kitchen chair with your feet on the floor and your spine held straight.
2 Take both arms out in front of you with the upper arms held parallel to the floor and both elbows bent at a right angle vertical to the floor.
3 Place your right arm over your left at the elbows so that the outer aspect of your arms touch each other.
4 Twine your forearms around each other so both palms are facing each other (albeit with the left palm lower down the forearm). Keep your upper arms held up parallel to the floor.
5 Now raise the whole tangled complex upwards, as high in front of your face as possible. You will feel a pulling sensation in your ribs where they attach to the spine in the upper back. The higher you go the more they will pull.
6 Hold for 15 seconds then relax.
7 Repeat three times then reverse the position of the arms and repeat another four times.

The thoracic side bend

This exercise helps flare the ribs apart at the front and the sides of the chest wall. It is especially useful when irritability of a spinal segment and its rib junctions has caused chronic spasm of the intercostal muscles. The tightness here causes the ribs to be held clutched together, almost lying along the top of one another, making it difficult for this band to expand enough to draw a deep breath. You invariably feel it easier to go one way than the other, but try to avoid bowing forward when stiffness of the lateral bend is encountered.

1 Sit towards the front of a chair with your feet on the floor and your spine held straight.
2 Bend each arm to a right angle, holding each elbow with your other hand.
3 Raise both arms above your head, pulling them right back beside your ears.
4 In this position bend your trunk sideways to the left, making sure you keep your upper arms in the same plane as your ears.
5 Hold the position for 15 seconds, breathing normally all the time, then release.
6 Repeat three more times to the left then change sides and do four times to the right.

Advanced

The twist on all fours

This exercise is particularly effective for a scoliotic spine. It is superbly effective at strengthening the small rotatores muscles between the thoracic segments, which give power to the twisting action in this part of the spine. Stretching the under hand along the floor helps free the ribs It is a very strenuous exercise and when doing the second part, care must be taken to get the upper arm right up to the vertical position. Make sure your hips and legs do not twist out of the pure kneeling stance.

1 Start on your hands and knees on the floor.
2 Turn your right hand palm-up with the fingers pointing trans-versely between your left hand and knee.
3 Let your right shoulder touch the floor as you bend the left elbow and slide your right hand between your left hand and knee as far as possible.
4 Firmly hold this hand on the floor and then pull back the upper shoulder slightly to complete the stretch. Hold the position for 10 seconds
5 Retract your right hand across the floor and take it in one sweep to above your head. It requires effort to keep your arm vertical.
6 Repeat once and then change sides and do it twice with the other hand.

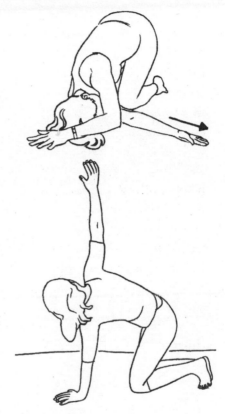

The plough

You will find the exercise difficult to do at first; it pulls on the neck, making it hard to breathe, but even holding it for a few seconds helps. You will feel a mixture of stretch and pain in your middle back which will be relieved by relaxing into the pain and gently breathing through it. The pose is good for people with a too-straight back. Bearing weight on the shoulders and the upper ribs gently forces the thoracic spine into a hoop, with a splaying out effect of the fish scales of the thoracic vertebrae. Rolling along your spine in the second part of the exercise is comforting for a very stiff thorax. It rhythmically releases the ribs as you roll over them and helps prise up recessed thoracic vertebrae. You often feel one side of the rib cage and certain ribs as more prominent and less yielding as you roll over them. This is an indication to stay there and mobilise them more by pivoting on them.

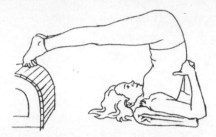

1 You will need a pillow and a small stool or low chair. Position the stool about 45 centimetres away from the pillow on the floor.
2 Lie on your back on the floor with the pillow positioned crossways under your shoulders and your head free on the floor. The pillow should be positioned to allow a step-down at the point where the thorax becomes the neck, and this spares the neck from too much pushing under. The more uncomfortable the neck feels, the higher the pillow step-down should be.
3 Raise both legs up and swing them over your head so the feet rest on the stool behind your head. Make this movement smooth not jerky.
4 Support your bottom with your hands (arms bent at the elbow) and hold this position for as long as you can—up to 2 minutes if possible—relaxed and breathing evenly all the time.
5 Keep your chin tucked in and roll down your thoracic spine. Remove the blanket and then roll back and forth several times on your upper back to simulate spinal rolling. Note: do *not* move your head while doing this exercise.

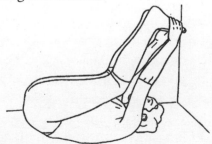

The thoracic BackBlock and angel's wings stretch

This is good for the round-shouldered back and is superbly effective for loosening tight ribs. It prises the segments straight by opening the fronts of your vertebral interspaces. It also pulls your ribs apart at the front, where they have collapsed down on one another and your intercostal muscles and soft tissues have tightened. The angel's wings in the second part of the exercise helps open the chest by stretching the pectoral muscles on the front of the shoulders and your chest wall. At the completion of this exercise you gain a real sense of being looser in your own skin and being able to walk tall.

1   Bend your knees as you lie on the floor and position the BackBlock underneath you on its flattest side, lengthwise. Use trial and error to position its top edge level with the base of your neck. Also take care to have it aligned straight down your spine.
2   Lie back on the BackBlock, then take your hands to your sides, and gently lower one leg at a time onto the floor.
3   Maintain this position for 2 minutes, doing minor adjustments to pull your chin in as you do.
4   To incorporate the arms in the stretch, take them over your head to rest them on the floor, fingers interlaced and palms turned away and your elbows straight. Your arms over your head like this often makes your neck feel more comfortable.

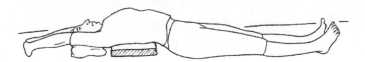

5   As you breathe out, take the arms in one sweeping semi-circular movement down to your sides, the backs of your hands in contact with the carpet all the way around. They will pass through a tighter, more uncomfortable arc in the top quadrant of the movement. Don't shirk this!

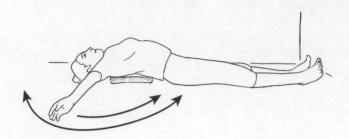

6   Rest at the bottom of the excursion and then breathe in as your arms go back up to the arms-above-your-head position. (It is okay to take another breath in and out before the return journey, if this makes you relax more.)

7   Repeat the angel's wings stretch twice, breathing slowly.

8   To come off the BackBlock, gently roll off to the side like a log, with your arms down.

Chapter three
Your neck

WHAT IS YOUR NECK?

Your neck is your spine's slender extension, emerging from your shoulders. Like so many other parts of the human body, your neck usually operates with such effortless grace that its highly sophisticated function can be overlooked. You can move it with spontaneous quick-starting action, despite carrying a heavy head, and stop it at will at any stage in its enormous range, at points calibrated to within fractions of degrees, so your senses can work optimally.

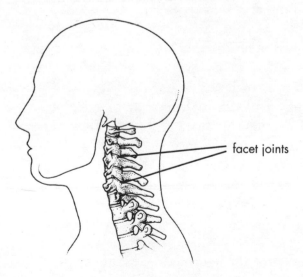

facet joints

FIGURE 3.1 The side view of the neck. The neck starts right up in the head.

Your neck is an exquisite though vulnerable piece of machinery; much more than a dancing column of bricks. Neuro-physiologically it is alive with nerve pathways, almost like an extension of the brain. A dense nervous lacework drapes itself over the jostling vertebral stack, threading through bony channels between the discs and facet joints. The nervous networks have many functions—some obvious, like supplying power to muscles and sensation to the skin of neck and arms; others subtle, like controlling primitive righting reflexes to coordinate balance, or the dilation of blood vessels to the brain. As we see elsewhere in the spine, the physical intimacy between your nerves and a free-wheeling mechanical structure is fraught with difficulty; even more so in your neck where the ana-tomy is so directly related to facilitating movement. This is never more obvious than when your neck starts going wrong. Then you see how directly limitation of movement and debility of function is associated with pain.

Whenever things in the neck go awry in a mechanical sense, the ill effects can be far-reaching and many-layered; some obvious, others diffuse and difficult to define. You will read later that apart from pain and stiffness of the neck, the disturbed functioning of your senses—often uniquely different with each sufferer—is the broad-brush picture of cervical dysfunction.

Clinicians confronted daily with a seemingly endless array of symptoms—from headache or migraine with blurred vision and spots before the eyes, to remorseless neck pain accompanied by a genuine lack of will to go on living—know well that much can be attributed to a neck being out of kilter. When the dysfunction of joints is dealt with and the neck runs true again, many of these symptoms simply fade away. It is a joy of our job; just one of the many.

Your neck consists of seven vertebrae, from the base of the skull to the top of the upper back. Each consists of a circular brick-like central body (vertebral body), two stunted wing-like projections either side (transverse processes), and one longer strut out the back (spinous process). As we have seen in the previous two chapters, the central bodies of the vertebrae are cushioned by the intervertebral discs. Once again, the discs act as fibrous links to attach the verte-brae and also as shock absorbers to cushion intervertebral contact.

Flanking the back of each disc, the vertebrae articulate above and below with their neighbours where the transverse processes notch together. These bone-to-bone junctions are known as the apophyseal, or facet joints.

Spinal nerve roots exit the spine in pairs, on left and right of the column, at the level of each intervertebral interspace. In leaving, they pass through a short bony canal (intervertebral foramen), which is bounded on one side by the intervertebral disc and the other by the facet joint. The nerve root is protected from the sucking and billowing machinery of these two working structures by a sleeve called the nerve sheath, like a shirtsleeve protecting the arm from a prickly coat. Even so, all spinal nerves leave the spine through the hinges of each spinal segment

Generous mobility—and the fact that it must be accurately controlled within range—is a big factor with necks. Neck mobility is directly related both to the fatness of its discs and the freedom of its facet joints. Although cervical discs are thinner in actual size than their lumbar brethren, they are massively thick in proportion to the height of their vertebrae. Thicker discs provide greater clearance between the vertebrae as they swivel about, making it easier for the facet joint surfaces to glance past one another as your neck turns.

Relative to vertebral size, cervical facet joints are much larger than elsewhere in your spine. Their big congruent dinner-plate surfaces, glistening with mother-of pearl cartilage, make for easy skidding contact. Their flatter orientation means the facets do not slot the spinal segments together as snugly as they do in the lower back, where bending must be powerfully restricted to be safe, though the large strong capsules of cervical facets adequately compensate for this.

There is one significant difference between vertebra-disc-vertebra unions in the neck compared to the rest of the spine. The vertebral bodies sweep up at the sides, making a bony rim top and bottom, which means that the discs themselves are virtually encapsulated by bone. These joints are called the joints of Luschka and their presence means that disc prolapse (where a degenerated disc material oozes out from between the bones and 'pinches a nerve') in the neck is extremely rare.

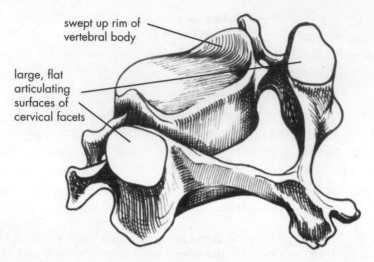

swept up rim of
vertebral body

large, flat
articulating
surfaces of
cervical facets

FIGURE 3.2 The swept-up rim of the vertebral rim makes cervical disc
prolapse rare.

HOW DOES YOUR NECK WORK?

The top two cervical vertebrae are different in many ways to the lower
five. The first vertebra—the atlas—articulates directly with the base of
the skull at the atlanto-occipital joint (C0–C1). Two rounded bumps
or condyles, on the base of the skull, like the rockers of a rocking
chair, fit exactly into two scooped-out hollows in the top of the atlas.
Thus the cranium rocks on the atlas, creating the nodding action of
the head. This action provides approximately 20 degrees of overall
neck flexion.

The second vertebra—the axis—is largely made up of one central
bony peg, which sticks up through a round central hole in the first
vertebra, like an index finger through a doughnut. This allows the
head and the first vertebra to spiral or axially rotate on the axis—at the
atlanto-axial joint (C1–C2) and it provides a large component of the
neck's twisting freedom.

Your neck has extraordinary mobility in all its ranges: rotation,
side flexing and the nodding and arching movements (flexion and
extension). Movement of your head utilises all three degrees of freedom, finely tuned as one. In different combinations you can put your

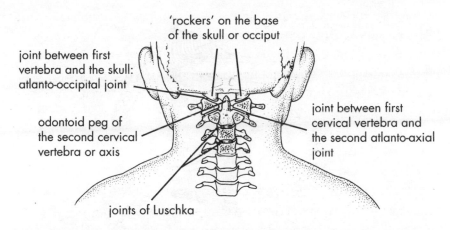

'rockers' on the base
of the skull or occiput

joint between first
vertebra and the skull:
atlanto-occipital joint

joint between first
cervical vertebra and
the second atlanto-axial
joint

odontoid peg of
the second cervical
vertebra or axis

joints of Luschka

FIGURE 3.3 Nodding happens at the atlanto-occipital joint (skull and first cervical vertebra) and swivel at the atlanto-axial joint (cervical 1 and 2).

face almost anywhere it wants to go: threading cotton through the eye of a needle, peering up at the undersurface of a table, or viewing the back of one's elbow.

Neck movement starts at T12, almost down at waist level, providing the essential background mobility for putting the head about. Thus the thorax sets the stage for your neck by positioning itself under where the head wants to go, like the puppeteer's gloved arm below the puppet's body. Without this mobile base, your neck would be a feeble swizzle stick, with tight jerky movements and a fraction of the range. It would also suffer immense strain at both ends, where it joins the solid block of the skull and where it plunges into the stiffer thorax.

Your neck spans thin air between the shoulders and skull like a delicate suspension bridge with muscles working all around it. Balancing your head atop this column while it moves is exacting, not the least because it requires seamless adjustments in muscle coordination and tone so your head doesn't shake or wobble. This is all the more difficult because a greater part of your head lies in front of the centre of gravity than behind it. The postural attitude of the neck plays a critical role in helping your neck muscles control your head's balance.

The flexors at the front of your neck draw the head forward and the chin down (perhaps their most arduous job of the day is lifting the head off the pillow in the morning), while the muscles at the back of your neck, the extensors, hold the head up. The flexors direct your head momentarily this way and that, whereas the extensors hold your head up there, waiting and prepared for movement as required. Neck extensors are on duty all our waking hours, preventing your head from flopping forward. They only go off duty when you sleep, which explains why your chin drops to your chest if you sleep sitting up. Immediately, you can see the disparity in workload between these two groups. And sure enough, their differing roles become distorted when your neck ceases to function well.

All your neck muscles work at slim margins of mechanical advantage and thus exert a downward compressive force upon your neck as they contract. A healthy arching of the neck (lordosis) helps ride out this compression, which a poker-straight neck will not do. The jaw projecting a greater distance in front of the column also makes the nodding-down action of the face easier, requiring less muscle effort. When the extensors pull the head back, the lordosis helps squelch the segments forward in a bowstring action, which also helps cervical discs escape direct vertical compression. You can see a similar thing in the lower back, where a heightened bowing forward of the lumbar spine on heel-strike helps soften the blow of impact during walking.

Finely honed head and neck control is always an elusive thing, especially since the muscles at the front of your neck commonly weaken, not unlike your tummy muscles in the lower back, and the muscles up the back of your neck commonly tighten (shorten). They will get tighter still if your neck joints are irritable, just as they do with heightened states of anxiety or fear.

Head and neck coordination through muscle control is also influenced by your arms, which hang heavily from the shoulders and tug laterally on your neck. You will read in the following chapter how dysfunctional use of the arms, which involves a hauling action of the shoulder forequarter, rather than a clean action at the ball and socket joint, can damage the cuff of the muscles wrapped around the top of your arms. This action also over-recruits your neck muscles to lift your arms and eventually it takes a toll on your neck. In the clinical forum this must be dealt with, though it may be difficult to say which problem came first, the neck or the arm—a neck problem causing weakness of the arms and making the shoulder action clumsy, or poor

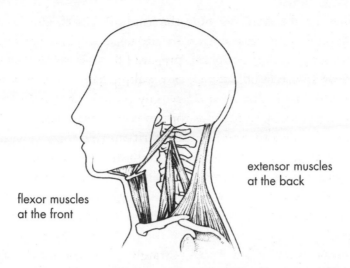

flexor muscles
at the front

extensor muscles
at the back

FIGURE 3.4 The angle pull of most of the neck muscles is very nearly
straight.

shoulder use (scapula stabilisation) causing a neck problem. In a typical chicken-and-egg syndrome it is important to address both ends of
the problem at once, irrespective of which is the primary complaint,
otherwise successful treatment won't happen.

This problem will get worse if your neck muscles go into guarding
mode as a reaction to your neck being thrown about by your arms.
The heightened tone of the clenched muscles compresses the cervical
joints, which racks up the pain cycle. The degree to which muscle
spasm heightens compression of spinal segments is difficult to
quantify (an area where researchers could greatly help clinicians!),
though experienced practitioners recognise spasm as an additional
pain source, making it difficult to set the neck free once it sets in.

The large quantity of fluid in the cervical discs helps your neck
absorb the weight of the super-heavy head (approximately 5 kilograms)
and imparts to it a floating quality as you move. Apart from helping to
keep your brain jangle free, the elastic sink-and-spring function of your
neck aids the free flow of blood up-hill to your brain through its
various cervical arteries. Your neck squashing down into a deeper
lordotic curve, followed by elastic recoil with the ebb and flow of
movement, also helps nourish the cervical discs. Fluid squeezed out
under the compression is replaced by a fresh quota, sucked back during

the upward release. This pump imbibition effect enhances fluid transfer and hence disc nutrition and thwarts discal breakdown. It provides ancillary dynamic pumping, which works mainly when you are active throughout the day, as distinct from the slower osmotic mechanism, which drags discal fluids in more slowly overnight.

Your neck's wide range of movement while supporting the weighty head makes it susceptible to incidental injury but postural attitude can set your neck up for strain in a more low-key way. In brief, necks that deviate from an optimal lordosis develop problems; too much lordosis almost as much as too little, though the provenance is different. Scoliosis lower down the spine also puts the neck out of balance.

WHAT ARE THE ACCESSORY MOVEMENTS OF YOUR NECK?

Neck movement involves a marked degree of twist so your head can turn easily at the command of your senses. Freedom of this top-heavy activity is kept in check by the bony hooking mechanism of the facet joints at each segmental level. Compared with the rest of the spine, the cervical facet joints are large shallow, scooped-out dinner plates. Their shape and flatter orientation encourages the upper vertebra to spiral around its neighbour below on highly polished, friction-free cartilage surfaces. As the top vertebra moves around, increasing tension of the tissues acts as a brake to provide another mechanism to keeping the stack of vertebrae taut and tightly held in place.

Facet control of your head's forward nodding works much as it does in the lower back to control bending. The lower facet surface slopes up at the front so that, during bending, the upper vertebra travels up-hill as it glides forward, thus increasing the tension of the restraining ligaments. In the mid-cervical spine, the steeper orientation of the facet makes the stop ramps steeper and therefore faster-acting, which is just as well since this is naturally a looser, more mobile part of the neck and thus the segments require greater holding as the neck bends. At the lower end of the neck, the facet surface stop ramps have a flatter orientation, which means the lower cervical facets naturally bear more load and the neck is naturally stiffer here.

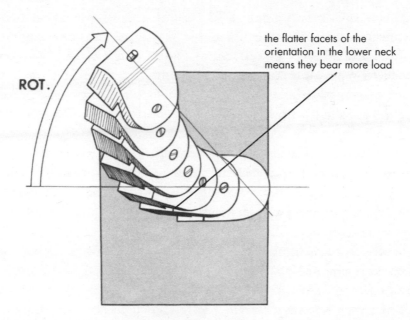

the flatter facets of the
orientation in the lower neck
means they bear more load

ROT.

FIGURE 3.5 The steeper orientation of mid-cervical facets helps control the head's nodding action in this 'looser' section of the neck.

Lower cervical stiffness is augmented by the criss-cross of muscles at the crossbar of the shoulders. Both factors go some way to explaining why arthritic change associated with disc thinning occurs most readily at low cervical levels (C5–6 and C6–7).

Facet joint freedom is the important accessory movement of the neck. Their orientation encourages both bending and twisting, without letting upper vertebrae slip off their lower kin. The right amount of accessory freedom is critical to necks feeling normal and working painlessly. Insufficient facet freedom restricts your neck's freedom, particularly when turning your head, whereas too much facet freedom, especially at the mid-cervical levels, can allow your neck to become over-mobile, though this may not be immediately obvious.

It is easy for experienced thumbs to palpate accessory freedom of your cervical facets. They form a chain down either side of the neck, just to the front of the thick cables of muscle, and when they are swollen they feel enlarged and sore to the touch. They are commonly mistaken for nodules. Palpation of a facet reveals how healthy it is.

If it is normal it feels empty, as if nothing is there—conspicuous by its inconspicuousness. When irritable, a facet is palpably thickened and its pressed-together surfaces will grind past one another when made to move. In the mid-cervical spine, facets can feel spongy or soggy—indicating hypermobility—which may cause other problems, especially if its partner above or below or on the other side is less mobile.

Palpating the facets also provides information about the joint capsules, thus revealing their degree of inflammation and whether the problem is acute or chronic. If the capsule is tense and leathery it indicates the problem is more longstanding. If it is bloated or doughy it is more recent.

Facet stiffness commonly causes pain and a host of other less specific symptoms but over-mobility of a facet may be elusive to pinpoint and harder to deal with. Tying up too-loose mid-cervical segments is not straightforward, though it usually requires loosening adjacent segments that are too stiff, particularly at the cervico-thoracic junction and the rest of the thoracic spine below.

Segmental freedom of the cervical vertebrae at the vertebra-disc-vertebra (known as the central core) is also an important accessory freedom for your neck. Poor mobility here in the forward/backwards gliding freedom is usually evident long before facet pathology is. Palpation of the spinous processes while you are in the prone position, with your forehead cupped in your hands, may reveal to the clinician stiffness to antero-posterior pressures at various cervical levels. Because of the inherent twisting freedom of your neck, axial rotation (evidenced by sideways movement of the spinous process) is another vitally important segmental movement.

Glitches in mobility between left and right axial rotation are very common at a segmental level and easily picked up through gauging transverse pressures to the spinous processes. Individual vertebrae frequently become stuck in a degree of axial rotation, so their 'tail' or spinous process sits to the left or right of midline and is stiff and painful to correct back to centre. The fixed axial twist tensions the diagonal lattice of the disc wall and introduces compression to the segment, further contributing to the immobility of that segment.

HOW DOES THE NECK GO WRONG?

Neck performance is very dependent upon optimal participation from the spine below, specifically the thorax. The reasons are related both to the posture and the mobility of the thorax, the latter usually being directly related to the former. When the thoracic spine fails to provide full background mobility, it seems all the natural features of your neck work against it—its fragility, the heaviness of your head and the imbalance of muscles controlling your head. Whatever the background cause, symptoms can arise from malfunction of either (or both) the two compartments of the cervical segment: the disc-vertebra component at the front or the facets at the back.

As we saw in chapter 1 on the low back, the outer layers of the disc walls are akin to a tension-resistant ligamentous skin and play a powerful role in binding your spinal segments together in a stack. This tensile outer skin is also the only part of the disc with a nerve supply. By contrast, the middle and inner disc walls behave more like a fluid-filled capsule to defray compression, and this part is not innervated. Postural stresses or outright accidental wrenching of a spinal segment can injure the outer disc wall, in exactly the way a ligament of your ankle can be strained. Ligamentous injury results in microscopic stretch and breakage of fibres, with subsequent loss of elasticity through scarring. The shortened ligament can then become painful because it has inadequate stretch to comply with normal movement demands. This is the fundamental pain of a stiff spinal segment.

Loss of disc compliance also minimises the sucking-and-blowing action of the secondary imbibition pump, so the disc struggles to nourish itself. Discs degenerate as a result of poor nutrition and as the disc gets drier, the process escalates. It also picks up apace as the shock absorption declines. As the fluid in the capsular part of the disc disappears it cannot keep your head afloat as effortlessly and the disc walls become the front line in shouldering axial load. The physical compression bunches down the disc's meshed walls and they traumatise as they are squashed more. Small pain receptors in the outer wall (mechano-receptors) start blitzing off messages about the jarring forces at work, adding another source of pain to a stiff link in your neck.

As discs lose vitality, they also lose the ability to pull apart with movement, so they begin to be assaulted by stretch as much as compression. Long before there is permanent disc thinning (visible on imaging) the segment may feel stiff when palpated from outside. To probing thumbs it feels like a plug of cement in a rubber hose. The cycle intensifies as ongoing trauma makes discs thinner. With increased load-bearing the walls become thicker and less elastic. In extreme cases the walls may calcify.

When the disc loses height, the syndrome of degeneration escalates as the facet surfaces at the corresponding level settle down in closer contact. This subjects the facets to extra load, which they are not designed to bear. The facets initially develop a low-grade inflammation in what is known as facet arthropathy but their loss of joint space also predisposes them to additional injury. The reduced clearance and room to move to ride out errant jinking can rattle the bony safety mechanism and lead to arthritic change of the joint.

Facet joints are the most easy to pull apart structures in your spine and a neck problem can be caused from an unlucky ricking incident that zeros in on a virgin joint, similar, though on a smaller scale, to twisting an ankle. But more usually, there is provenance of subclinical drying and thinning of the intervertebral disc, thus putting the facet next in line for injury.

When the facet is the originating problem, breakdown of the entire segment can work in reverse order. The resulting muscle spasm protecting the inflamed facet screws down the segment, like the corner wing nuts on a flower press squashing the surfaces shut. This makes the whole vertebra stiffer in the column, causing a secondary stiff spinal segment.

Facet joints are highly sensitive to malfunction and are much keener to register pain than discs. A highly sophisticated nerve supply, coupled with extreme vascularity (blood supply) make facet capsules ready to pick up and react to abnormal stresses. Even minor mechanical duress is felt as discomfort. Their labile response causes local tenderness and aching soreness in the side of your neck, shoulder or upper arm (depending on the facet level). The soreness in the side of your neck typically craves rubbing and squeezing and digging in with the fingers.

More severe facet irritation invokes protective guarding of your neck muscles, which in turn causes bloating compression of the facet and inflames it more. As discussed, spasm in the spine can be the wild card that transforms a nuisance niggle into a nightmare neck. Spasm can be felt as tension in your neck and across the top of your shoulders with the tone so hard it invites pummelling with an iron bar. It is painful in a twinging dull way but, more significantly, it makes your neck move discordantly, thereby fueling the original problem and making it worse. This is particularly so if raised tone (spasm) is evident in some muscles but not others; at the back of your neck but not the front, or restricted to one side only, as if some strings of a puppet are pulled too tight.

Disturbed muscle tone upsets the subtle way your neck operates, with its invisible baton changes as one muscle lets go and another takes over. Fluent seamless coordination is lost, as the raised tone elevates the threshold before a muscle automatically switches off. When this over-active group fails to let go on cue, your neck can jar painfully as it goes to move. An agonising jolt can rip through your neck, which is unnervingly painful and encourages any future movement to be undertaken much more cautiously.

A similar jolting muscle clench can happen if your neck remains too long in one position—head down typing, or turned one way looking at a television. Your neck cranks to start and judders to a stop and the head seems too heavy for the shoulders. Folding your arms across the chest relieves the dragging down tension on the side neck muscles. Pummelling the tense marbles of the swollen capsules in the neck gives temporary relief but pain will soon return.

Anxiety and fear can make muscle-guarding keep on keeping on. Your neck will become even more tense, overlaying the pre-existing automatic tension with additional volitional guarding. Minus the light and shade of the normal on–off movement, blood flow dams up in the locked-away problem joint. In extreme cases, bloating of an inflamed facet can impinge on the nerve root where it exits the spine close by. Thus, the nerve itself inflames, in what is known as neuritis or a pinched nerve (*see* below). Fully blown neuritis is rare. Much more common is an achy joint in your neck, which refers pain to your arm.

Disturbances of spinal alignment can predispose cervical segments to both facet joint arthropathy and stiff spinal segment. When your thoracic spine is too straight, the neck usually continues on too straight above it. The cervical segments sit vertically atop one another and weight through your neck is borne directly by the discs, instead of sharing it with the facets at the back. This creates a pile-driving effect as the discs suffer direct-hit vertical compression during weight-bearing. Many levels in your neck will become stiff spinal segments as they lose fluid and thud on impact. They may develop secondary facet arthropathy, eventually, as disc thinning lets the tyre down, so to speak, and causes the facets to bear excess load.

With a too-hunched thoracic spine, neck problems accrue for different reasons. A too-rounded upper back projects your neck forward at an angle, making it necessary to over-arch back again (extreme lordosis) to get your eyes looking straight ahead, not at the floor. The head carried this far in front of the line of gravity also invokes excessive restraint from the facets of your lower neck to stop the segments shearing forward off one another. Here your neck literally hangs on its facets.

Long-acting postural strain of the muscles at the back of your neck also plays a role in this syndrome. The upper fibres of upper trapezius, which fan out from the base of the skull to the tips of the shoulders, must work overtime to pull the head back over the rest of the column. This is a heavy muscular workload and the over-activity of trapezius sometimes creates a permanent webbing-up across the angle between neck and shoulder.

Fibrositis may develop in trapezius fibres from the postural strain. Fibrositis is thought to be a clumping together of muscle fibres and alteration of anatomical structure through over-contraction. This may be palpable with the fingers as painful ropey cords at the back of your neck/shoulder.

Over-activity of upper trapezius can perpetuate neck problems by causing reciprocal under-activity of lower trapezius. This leads to poor stabilisation of your shoulder blades (scapulae), making them poke out from the back of the chest wall, like embryonic wings. This adds to the stoop of your shoulders and makes it harder for the neck to attain an upright, more anatomically pleasing posture. As you will read in the following chapter, poor scapula stability is usually the

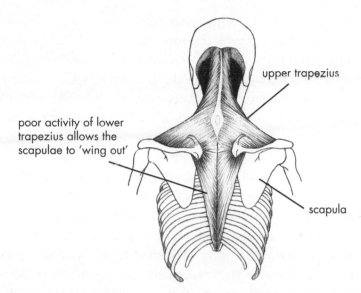

upper trapezius

poor activity of lower
trapezius allows the
scapulae to 'wing out'

scapula

FIGURE 3.6 Upper trapezius is often overactive when lower trapezius is
underactive.

cause of shoulder trouble, which explains why a stooped thoracic
posture, weak tummy and sway neck often occur hand in glove with
shoulder problems.

Both the forced facet engagement and static clenching of trapezius
telescope the lower cervical segments together, making the base of the
neck stiffer. The compression affects both the central core (vertebra-
disc-vertebra) and the facets. Commonly, the mid-cervical segments
become over-mobile to compensate for lack of movement lower down.
As the condition becomes more complex, the under-mobile segments
tend to perpetuate the existence of the over-mobile ones, and vice versa.

It is easy for therapists to feel stiff segments with the patient lying
prone, forehead cupped in the palms and head in mid position. The
spinous processes usually sit up proud of the others and are stiffer
and painful to depress. Stiff and over-mobile segments co-existing
side by side can make your neck feel very wonky and headaches are a
common feature of this problem. Initially, it may be hard to know if
pain is coming from the loose or the stiff segments, or indeed whether
the mobility problem is of the facets or the central core. Whatever the
diagnosis, treatment often requires dealing with the posture and
freedom of the thoracic spine initially for therapy to be effective.

Spinal scoliosis is lateral-twisting curvature through the spine, visible when viewed from behind, which may be acquired congenitally or through a shorter leg. When it is acquired through leg-length difference, the sacrum tilts down to the side of the shorter leg, causing the spine to compensate back and forth all the way up, so the head can balance at the top. The natural laxity of the neck's facet joints allows important adjustments for anomalies of curve further down, primarily so the eyes can operate on the same plane to focus and judge distance. A permanent twisted sit of your neck will take a toll on your neck joints.

When your spine bends laterally the segments twist on their axes, which closes the facets on one side and pulls them open on the other. Indefinite compression or tension of the highly electrified facets eventually causes secondary inflammatory arthropathy, though the dynamics of strain are different. The close-packed facet will be the first to suffer cartilage breakdown and the pulled apart one will develop capsular irritation, though it is never possible to say which will cause symptoms first.

Lateral curvature pinches the vertebra at the apex centrally at the inter-body joint (vertebra-disc-vertebra) making it a stiff spinal segment. This vertebra often sits recessed deeper than the others, like a piano key that won't come up, and even experienced hands find it difficult to prise free.

THE COMMON DISORDERS OF THE NECK

Segmental stiffness of the cervical spine

Injury to your neck can take place in a variety of ways, either as a shunting-twisting strain across the column, or as vertical compression. Being stretch-sensitive, the outer disc wall is vulnerable to both transverse shunting injuries and sustained postural strains. Even small jarring incidents, while lifting say, may target one disc, simply by the luck of the draw, and cause microscopic over-stretching of its outer wall fibres. The vertebrae then stick together at the central core, like cotton reels glued together. Sluggish fluid exchange through the disc causes a build-up in metabolites and a painful unease is felt throughout your whole neck, thus roping in the healthy levels and making them uncomfortably stiff too.

Stasis of circulation, coupled with tension of your neck muscles, makes your neck feel like a poker, inviting extremes of arching movement to make it run freer. Your neck will feel looser and the head lighter for a brief period but, sooner than later, it tightens up again and needs releasing. Some people get hooked on clicking—or self-manipulating. Though this may make their neck feel better in the short term, in the long term it causes progressive scarring of the facet capsules and makes the problem segment more bound up. You will learn later in the self-help section how sustained stretching is much more effective than wrenching the neck harder and harder to achieve that elusive click.

Manual investigation by a trained therapist is the most accurate method of gauging a problem. More importantly, it reveals specifically the direction of restricted mobility. Having the problem levels touched is often a relief; a sweet pain, as if the troublemaker has been rumbled. As with other parts of your spine, the stiff link usually feels as if the bone itself is bruised. This may not correspond to the level that looks the worst on the scans—remember scans and X-rays do not show stiffness any more than a photograph reveals a rusty hinge of a door. Remember too that imaging of all kinds invariably highlights the unimportant and overlooks the critical issue.

Your discomfort will wax and wane, though you are usually hard pressed to pinpoint the nub of things and the actual problem level. The muscles in spasm can make your neck seem thicker and a typical sign of trouble is difficulty doing up the top button of a shirt. In its lesser moments your neck will be stiff more than sore, though it never feels quite right. The pain is often described as gnawing and tiring and the head too heavy for the shoulders.

Excessive muscle tone of your cervical extensors also increases vertical compression of your neck and reduces clearance between the vertebrae. This may account for the common finding of multiple segments fixed off-centre in minute but significant degrees of axial rotation. The clamping-down may cause the vertebrae to jink imperceptibly this way and that, like a stack of dinner plates slipping askew while being carried. The vertebrae assume a higgledy-piggledy alignment with their spinous processes stuck either side of the midline and painful to manual correction.

It is very important to correct the misalignment with physical treatment (using transverse pressures with the thumbs) in addition to releasing the forwards and backwards freedom of the jammed segment (P-A pressures). Being twisted off-centre laterally stretches the lattice of the disc wall, adding an extra component of compression to the segment, rather like a screw-top lid on a jar clamping it down tight.

Eventually a stiff spinal segment will be detectable on X-rays as a thinner disc, although there may be years of pain before this becomes evident. As we saw in chapter 1 on the low back, a segment sitting on a thinner disc harbours a propensity to eventually become hypermobile, simply because its reduced water content reduces the tensile strength of the spinal link. The ligaments spanning the narrowed interspace pucker, as does the flaccid disc wall. The tensile strength of the segment as a whole is then reduced, thereby jeopardising its security in the stack.

In some instances, perhaps related to a neck-jerking incident, the segment that seemed unbudgeable is knocked loose. Alternatively, hypermobility may develop by attrition as the low-pressure link is progressively stretched and weakened by activity. X-rays and scans at this stage reveal tooth-like projections of bone (osteophytes) at the interface between vertebral body and disc.

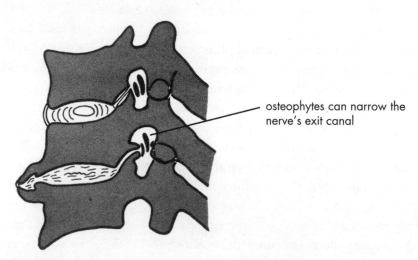

osteophytes can narrow the nerve's exit canal

FIGURE 3.7 Bony outgrowth (osteophytes) around the vertebral body and/or facet joints indicate past or current instability.

Though perhaps unsightly, osteophytes are important telltale signs that a segment is, or has been, hypermobile. They are thought to be the body's natural way of throwing out extra bone to stabilise a loose vertebra. Osteophytes are often described as bony spurs and blamed for piercing nerves causing pain, particularly arm pain. This over-simplistic rationale for surgical intervention is not good practice. Spurs are in no way a source of pain and do not require removal simply because they are there. It's the underlying cause of the spurs that needs attention.

Chronic facet joint arthropathy

Chronic facet joint arthropathy commonly follows on from a stiff spinal segment. Disc thinning causes lowered clearance between the vertebrae and forces contact between the facet surfaces. It is not possible to establish why, for example, a left in preference to a right facet is annoyed, though mild scoliosis and minute leg-length difference may have a role to play. The facet most subject to wear will gradually become stiffer. As its function closes down, movement demand can be shunted elsewhere—perhaps across to its corresponding partner on the other side, or to a level above or below. This explains the diagonal criss-cross siting of inflamed facets from one side to the other, all the way up through the neck as the problem snowballs.

With thinning of the discal pillow the joint space narrows and the facet capsule shrinks. With less room to move the surfaces abrade off a fine spume of cartilage dust, which silts up the joint. Fragments of cartilage act like a pot-scourer, stimulating quantities of lubricating fluid to sluice the chafing surfaces clean. As an ongoing process, large (macrophage) cells in the synovial fluid systematically devour bits of floating cartilage debris to keep the joint surfaces running freely.

Excess synovial fluid trapped in a joint causes problems as the inner capsular lining is inflamed by being stretched. The tensely swollen joint then limits movement, provoking acute shrieks of pain whenever unguarded movement squashes its very bulk. Your neck will be reluctant to move and loath to go in all its painful directions, either to squash or stretch a joint.

As your neck loses mobility, poor stretch of the facet capsules causes trauma, which is a source of secondary degeneration. Unselfconscious movement of your neck may unwittingly tug at tightened facet capsules as your head attempts to keep up with normal demands. Routine activity pings capsular fibres—either stretching or breaking them on a microscopic scale—at various levels. Scar tissue infiltrates the capsule as the fibres are repaired, ultimately making it tighter and even less accepting of stretch. Thus the degenerative process steps up a notch or two. As the strain tells, discord is sprayed around everywhere and, increment by increment, the problem becomes more widespread. It will become harder to keep your head moving with effortless ease. Harder to turn your head, and harder, for instance, to reverse the car out of the driveway!

The source of pain from facet arthropathy is threefold: local tenderness of the malfunctioning joint, referred pain and muscle spasm. Actual joint pain is localised to the side of your neck and often locatable to the exact level with your finger tips. The joint capsule feels swollen and tense, like a painful marble and it often craves direct pummelling from the hands.

Referred pain is not the same thing. It is a vague ache with ill-defined boundaries, extending into your arms and upper back, to areas which use the same nerve supply—similar to the way the pain of a heart attack is felt in the left arm. A parallel mechanism also results in referred tenderness, where the area becomes sore to the touch. Referred pain is much more diffuse than direct irritation of the nerve itself (*see* below) and it not directly affected by neck movement.

In less acute conditions, your neck will simply feel stiff and achy with grating noises during movement, like sand in the cogs, from the facet surfaces scraping. Patients with a stiff neck sense the first signs of old age as the head won't twist freely and the whole body must turn to help it. In its more advanced stages your neck will be locked in perpetual high-pitched pain, which screeches more if the neck is jerked.

As well as neck pain, degeneration of the cervical facets causes a host of other symptoms, not easily defined but related to cerebral function. These are often difficult to qualify, though patients know when their necks are bad because they don't feel quite right or 'with it'. They often feel dissociated from their own body, as if seeing life through a skein of gauze, and this often coincides with nausea, headache and inability to concentrate.

Although pain eventually becomes paramount, the more ethereal symptoms can be almost as unwelcome. Poor sleep quality may be a feature of cervical arthropathy and this may contribute to the commonly observed symptoms of anxiety and depression, unstable emotions, dizziness, ringing in the ears, disturbed hearing, blurred vision, difficulty swallowing, sinusitis or painful teeth … just to mention a few.

Acute wry neck

This is usually the result of a jolt or minor injury to your neck and may not have its beginnings in previous segmental stiffness. The facet joints are naturally looser and easier to pull apart than the cotton-reel junctions of the vertebral bodies sitting on their discs. This problem usually starts life as a mishap, a chance awkward movement that strains a healthy facet in preference to the disc—swinging at a golf ball that doesn't connect, turning to look behind you as you go down a step, or it may even be the unwelcome event of whiplash from a car accident. On the other hand, it can be something much more subtle, like falling asleep with the neck at an angle.

Acute wry neck can also start life as an acute facet-locking incident. This usually takes the form of a fluke, incidental movement that sneaks under the guard of the postural mechanisms and catches the stabilising structures of the neck unawares. The unexpected movement is always trivial; a minor glitch in streamlined movement which unluckily disjoints one facet. Before the muscles can react in time to control it, this tiny errant movement allows the congruent joint surfaces to slip slightly askew. The muscles then over-react, too late and with excessive gusto, with an excruciating jolt of spasm that locks the local link out of joint and jams the neck rigid.

The slight slippage (subluxation as distinct from dislocation) strains the joint at the centre of things and the ligaments are tugged. The usual process of inflammation ensues: effusion of fluid—and, if severe enough, blood—into the tissues around the joint, which stays there and solidifies into scar tissue. The most difficult manifestation is the guarding of the muscles, making your neck rigid and exquisitely painful to move.

Acute wry neck is painfully worrying and feels as if the neck is stuck out of joint. The muscles of the side of your neck stand up like ropes, with your head cocked awkwardly at an angle. All your movements will be guarded and painful, especially if your neck is jerked. Being a passenger in a car that rapidly accelerates can be agonising. Unlike chronic neck problems, which cause a low-grade, aching tension of the muscles at the back of the neck, acute arthropathy causes protective spasm of the muscles at the front and sides of the neck. Sudden movements cause a shriek of pain as the front and side muscles contract.

At the height of the crisis all your movements will be restricted, though doing them slowly, to avoid invoking a protective response often reveals you have a greater range than initially thought. Turning your head over on a pillow during the night may involve levering your whole body over while holding your head. Getting up in the morning may be the most painful event of the day and it may even be necessary to lift your head by pulling your hair. Sometimes it is possible to bring about a miraculous recovery by manipulating the locked joint—if you can get to the physio/osteopath/chiropractor before the muscle spasm sets in. A finely executed manipulative thrust in the right direction, can open the joint and let it slot back together in correct anatomical alignment, thus allowing you to walk away on air. More usually though, it needs several days of painkillers, anti-inflammatory drugs and muscle relaxants before it is possible to sneak in under the guard of the muscles and manipulate it free.

Invariably, a jammed joint needs preparatory mobilising—using thumb pressures to prise the vertebra free—before it is suitable for manipulative release. Even without manipulation, the slower method of mobilising will achieve the same result, and be more thorough in the long-term. As the clench of the joint releases, the natural congruency of the opposing joint surfaces encourages them to creep back into proper alignment. This approach is ideal for patients who are afraid of cervical manipulation.

Whatever the treatment, it is critically important to finally clear the joint by manipulation; otherwise the neck retains vestiges of a link caught-up inside, which can go on to seed future trouble in the form of chronic facet joint arthropathy. These are the necks that are never the same again after an original locking incident.

Acute brachial neuralgia

If an acute facet arthropathy does not subside within a relatively short period (two to three weeks), the intense local inflammation may cause oozing of toxic exudates from the exterior of the highly vascular joint capsule. This creates sticky adhesions that occupy valuable space in the nerve's already tight exit canal. Adhesions solidifying with age can embed the nearby spinal nerve in scar tissue, thus tethering the root and its sleeve to the capsule. Another unwanted wrench that hits the previously inflamed cervical facet precisely can tweak the nerve root, where it is bound down, and create an additional site of inflammatory reaction.

Nervous tissue is more sensitive to stretch than it is to cutting, pulverising and even burning and a spinal nerve can be greatly irritated by a local yanking trauma, even on a small scale. The nerve itself can become inflamed (neuritis) and may go on to become the source of agonising pain down the arm or deep into the shoulder.

With brachial neuralgia there is usually little pain in the neck and patients are often downcast that some trivial action, which invariably they cannot recall, could be the source of such strife. Patients often relate that prior to the full-blown flare-up they felt warnings from their neck if they made a sudden move. Throwing something light, like a sock for example, at an awkward angle could feel as if their arm did not have adequate give to let fly. The culprit action was barely worthy of comment but it may have managed to be in the specific direction to pull at tethered nerve fibres where they were bound down. The pain usually comes on slowly as an ache and feels like a strained muscle. It relentlessly builds to a crescendo through the arm and patients often note, barely in jest, that they would like the arm chopped off!

The pain of brachial neuralgia is typically described as unbearable nerve pain and, depending on which root is involved, is felt in different locations in the arm. It can be a breathtakingly nasty pain, often described as 'lancinating' (piercing) in jagged shards through the arm. The pain may also manifest in flooding fiery waves down the arm whenever the neck is moved to impinge the swollen facet on the nerve. Moving the arm in a way that stretches the inflamed nerve also provokes pain. The slightest increase in tension sets it off, making it difficult to find a comfortable position. Sometimes the arm is only pain-free with the hand on top of the head. This is known as the antalgic posture and it relieves pain by taking the nerve fully off the stretch. People can sit for hours cradling their arm.

When physical pressure builds up in the engorged joint the normal access and egress of cleansing blood slows to a sluggish trickle. The circulation dams up and the joint becomes more bloated, angry and inflamed. Its very own distension locks it out of movement within the neck's normal machinery. The repair process is hampered.

Physical treatment is aimed at probing the joint gently with the thumbs to dissipate engorgement and get the locked link into action. It is sometimes difficult to get this happening without invoking a painful treatment reaction and medication is usually needed to cover early treatment sessions. Anti-inflammatory drugs and muscle relaxants allow the swelling to seep away and painkillers give a much needed holiday from the pain because, remember, pain makes pain.

Sometimes a nerve root distended around the swollen bulk of a bulging intervertebral disc brings about the stretching of the nerve but in my experience this is rare, certainly in the neck. Disc bulges here are uncommon because the joints of Luschka fairly well contain the disc. It is also true that disc bulges anywhere in the spine are more inert and less bloody affairs than highly inflamed facet joints and therefore less likely to be implicated in limb pain.

Discs themselves do not have a blood supply. The fibro-elastic disc material, even when a bulge distends the innervated outer wall, is like fingernail and remains relatively aloof from rabid inflammation. Not so with an inflamed facet joint. By contrast it is red, irritable and swollen, like an inflamed sore throat. In terms of its effect on the spinal nerve, this combination of friction, stretch and inflammation is a potent source of trouble.

WHAT CAN YOU DO ABOUT IT?

The cases outlined above are the extremes. One hopes to catch these problems when the mechanical cause is still in its infancy. The way to thwart the problem in the first place, or rectify it if it has gone beyond that point, is to recapture a proper working dynamic between your neck and its mobile base. This means that your thorax must have as near-as-possible perfect postural alignment and also be fully mobile, both at its intervertebral and costo-vertebral joints (where the ribs meet the spine).

The base of your neck marks an abrupt functional transition from the fairly stiff casement of your thorax to your freewheeling elongated neck. In effect, the upper end of the column is like a slender spinal stalk emerging from the thorax, like a tortoise peering out of its shell. In other respects, the transverse line across your shoulders is like a crossbar on a ship's mast and, correspondingly, the musculature that binds the shoulder girdle to the cervico-thoracic junction is inordinately strong. Your shoulder girdle is like a weighty coathanger, lashing itself to the spine to give anchorage to your arms. All this can make the angle between your neck and shoulders a very bunched-up area, especially if anxiety and tension are part of everyday life. Since neck function is so reliant upon optimum contribution from the thoracic spine, from down as far as T12, it is critically important that the criss-cross of muscles at the base of your neck does not choke your neck off from movement of its mobile base.

Beginners

The head clasp

This exercise gently stretches the muscles down the side of the neck, which tend to shorten when your neck is held immobile by muscle spasm. When one side of your neck is shorter it holds that shoulder higher. This is not a very comfortable exercise and the range of movement achieved is small. You will often find your neck will go to one side more easily and that the stiffer side bends with a dog-leg rather than a free-flowing lateral curve.

1 Sit evenly on a chair with your feet comfortably flat on the floor in front of you.

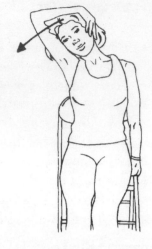

2 Place your left hand, palm down, under your left buttock so you are sitting on it.
3 Tilt (not turn) your head to the right.
4 Bring your right hand up and over your head. Spread the fingers of your right hand wide and cup the left side of the face as far down as you can reach. The weight of your right forearm will be along the upper-left aspect of your crown, reinforcing the right angulation of the head.
5 Hold for 15 seconds and release.
6 Repeat twice and then change sides, to stretch the other side of the neck three times.

The elbow lift

This exercise emphasises the backward movement of your head and neck on your shoulders, so it is effectively the counter-posture to all those hours spent with the head bent forward, focusing on a small field of vision. The movement should accentuate taking your neck back on your thorax, rather than simply tipping your head back at the top of your neck. When you take your neck right back you feel activity as far down as the mid-back, almost at waist level, though you can make the stretch less taxing by not taking your elbows so high and your chin so far back.

1 Stand with your feet squarely on the floor and clasp your hands together, intertwining your fingers.
2 Place your clasped hands under your jaw so as little as possible of the hands protrudes past the line of your chin and pinch your elbows together.
3 Keeping your elbows pinned together, raise their tips in an arc away from your chest and point them towards the ceiling, inhaling

as you go. This action tips your head back on your shoulders. Your fists reinforce the backwards angulation of both head on neck and neck on thorax.

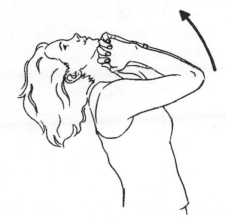

4 Relax and bring your elbows back down to your chest, exhaling as you go.

5 Repeat three times.

Intermediate

The plough extender

This exercise loosens an immobile thoracic spine, providing greater mobility for your neck's base to help share movement strain. The second part of the exercise stretches the extensor muscles down the back of your neck which habitually shorten in the presence of chronic muscle spasm. You will need a folded blanket or pillow and a low stool.

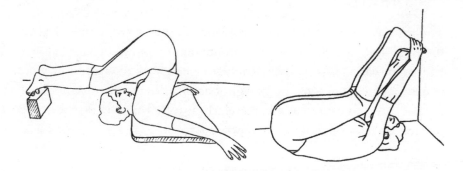

1 Put the stool about 45 centimetres away from your folded blanket or pillow on the floor.

2 Lie on your back, positioning your shoulders on the folded blanket with the stool beyond your head, not near your feet. The blanket should be placed to allow a step-down at the point where your thorax becomes your neck; this allows your neck to float

freely and spares it from too much pushing under during the exercise. The more uncomfortable your neck feels, the higher the blanket step-down needs to be made.

3   Raise both legs up and swing them over your head so your feet rest on the stool behind your head, supporting your bottom with your hands (arms bent at the elbows). Make sure the movement of swinging your legs over is smooth not jerky.

4   Hold this position for as long as you can—up to 2 minutes if possible—relaxed and breathing evenly all the time. You will feel a mixture of stretch and pain in your middle back, which will be relieved only by relaxing into the pain and gently breathing through it.

5   Keep your chin tucked in, roll down slowly, either completely or part-way. Roll back up into the pose.

6   Roll back and forth along the thoracic spine several times. As you get more adept at the rolling, the spine will loosen and you will find you can progress the posture further by removing the stool and allowing your knees to bend down towards your forehead. Once there you can rest for 30 seconds, gently breathing through the pain to achieve relaxation.

The swastika

This exercise is the most effective way of restoring the ability of your neck to twist. As your head turns to the right it puts the facets down the right side of your neck into a close-packed position, which disperses swelling from the joint capsules, a bit like wringing out a dishcloth. At the same time it stretches the joint capsules on the other side of the neck by pulling the facets apart.

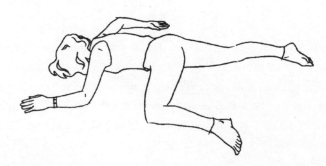

1 Lie on your front on the floor with your head turned to the right.
2 Bring your left arm out at 90 degrees and then bend your left elbow at a right angle so the palm of your hand on the floor is above your head.
3 Bring your right arm out to make a right angle with your shoulder and also bend that elbow at 90 degrees but this time downwards, so the palm faces upwards and rests out by your right hip. Your left arm will be crooked up and rotated externally; your right arm will be crooked down and rotated internally.
4 Bring your left leg so the upper leg is at 90 degrees to the body and the knee is bent to a right angle. The right leg remains straight on the floor.
5 Hold this position for at least 2 minutes. You will feel a stretch all through your neck and across your shoulders into your upper torso.
6 Periodically lift your head and move your cheek further away from your left arm, making it flatter on the floor. This is quite a stretch.
7 Change sides and repeat the exercise in the opposite direction. Make sure your head is always turned towards the hand you cannot see.

Advanced

The kneeling neck twist

This posture is a progression of the previous and it targets the facets at the base of your neck. As it puts your neck into a full twist, it also pushes it back on the thorax, so you feel a sensation of discomfort where the upper ribs join the spine. To maximise the stretch, lift your thighs up to an almost vertical position, which pushes your cheek more onto the floor.

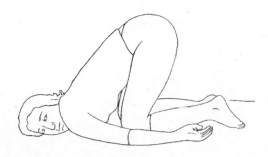

1 Kneeling on your hands and knees, release your arms so the right side of your face is resting with one cheek on the floor. You can lessen the stretch by lowering your bottom closer to your heels but the higher your bottom the greater the stretch and benefit.

2 One by one, slowly place your arms by your sides and hold the position for one minute, breathing gently. You can place your hands beside your face to lessen the pressure on your cheek if you feel the need.

3 To withdraw, bring your arms up one at a time and lift the weight off your neck.

4 Lower yourself again and turn your face to the other cheek. Repeat once in both directions.

Headstand

Yoga aficionados say inverted postures (at least 3 minutes per day) keep the brain clear, prevent hardening of the arteries and encourage collateral circulation through the brain. But headstands are not for everyone because it literally means taking most of your weight through your neck. Weight bearing through the crown puts extreme pressure changes on the cervical facets, and that stimulates cartilage regeneration of the joint surfaces. The posture invokes a strong co-contraction of both the flexor and extensor muscles and makes the neck considerably stronger and more erect. Extra strength allows the neck to resist the tendency to bow forward and shrink down into the shoulders; that sure sign of encroaching age. The exercise is particularly beneficial for necks that grate loudly when you turn

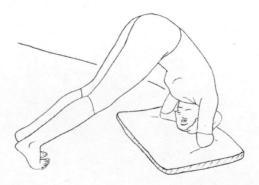

your head (crepitus), though it should always be undertaken with care and the neck should never be moved while you are in position.

1   Place a folded blanket in front of a wall.
2   Kneeling in front of the wall, interlace your fingers and make a 'V' with your forearms on the floor just wide enough to place the crown of your head on the blanket in between.
3   Straighten your legs as you take weight on your head on the floor, and then kick up with one leg first.
4   After both legs are vertical, take as much weight through your forearms as possible, making your neck long and your body as straight and light as possible.
5   While in position, keep your eyes open and continue pushing up through your neck and body to lessen cervical compression. This means hard work for your arms and shoulders.

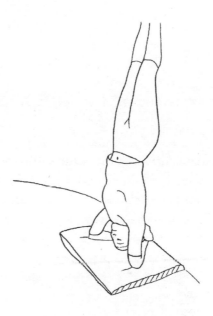

6   Remain in position for up to 3 minutes (although initially you will manage only a few seconds).
7   Do not repeat until your next exercise session.

Chapter four

Your shoulders

WHAT IS YOUR SHOULDER?

The shoulder joint is made where your arm joins your torso. It is a very mobile joint, which allows multi-directional freedom of your arm. In theory it is a ball-and-socket joint, though in practice it is hardly that. The ball is there all right; a large round knob, about the size and shape of an ice-cream on a cone at the top of the long shaft of the upper arm, the humerus. But the arm socket bears little resemblance to its counterpart in the hip. Instead of being a deeply-set bony pocket which encapsulates the ball, as the socket in the pelvis does the head of thigh bone (femur), the socket of the shoulder joint is a shallow little saucer.

The arm socket (the glenoid cavity) projects off the side of the shoulder blade (scapula) and is about the size of a scooped out twenty-cent piece. The round head of the humerus hangs gently against this socket, and skids around on it as your arm moves. The muscles which work your upper arm thread around the humeral head and help hold your arm in the socket. Collectively they are known as the rotator cuff muscles. They reinforce the baggy shoulder joint capsule in holding the shoulder together. Thus your arm hangs loosely off the shoulder girdle, like a coat sleeve dangling from a coathanger.

Above the humeral head is a bony ledge made by the collar bone (the clavicle) at the front and the bony ridge (the spine) of the scapula at the back. At the shoulder tip, these two bones form a union called

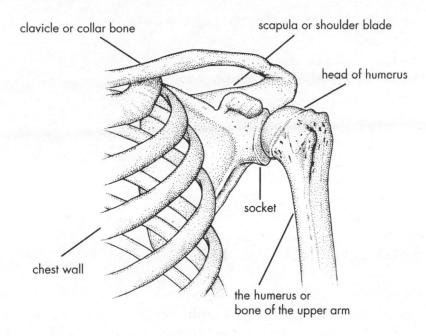

clavicle or collar bone

scapula or shoulder blade

head of humerus

socket

chest wall

the humerus or
bone of the upper arm

FIGURE 4.1 **The arm hangs off the shoulder like a sleeve off a coat-hanger.**

the acromio-clavicular joint. This joint creates a slight hood over the head of the humerus, which affords some stability for your shoulder, especially during the movement of lifting your arm over your head. However, the acromio-clavicular joint can be ruptured by violent upwards force along the shaft of the humerus, such as suffered when falling on the outstretched arm.

In a more subtle though similar way, you will see that dysfunctional use of your arm over a period of time can cause fraying of some of the muscle tendons where they loop over the top of the humeral head. The alarm roused by this process causes the plait of muscles holding the ball against the socket to go into guarding mode, which amounts to a whole-scale protective clench of all the muscles encompassing this joint. In itself this can be painful and further restricts the freedom of your shoulder movement—and if your luck is out—may go on to become fully fledged frozen shoulder.

HOW DOES YOUR SHOULDER WORK?

The arm joins to the torso at the glenoid cavity of the scapula, but the scapula itself is not a rigid fixture. It has its own movement, which supplies another dimension of freedom in putting your arm about. Scapula involvement profoundly enhances the dexterity of your hand. If you then add the usefulness of your opposing thumb, you see why the upper limb is so devastatingly effective at precision work and manipulating objects. The source of this brilliant mechanism however owes itself to two main factors: the sloppy utility of the shoulder joint and the background ability of the scapula to put itself in position.

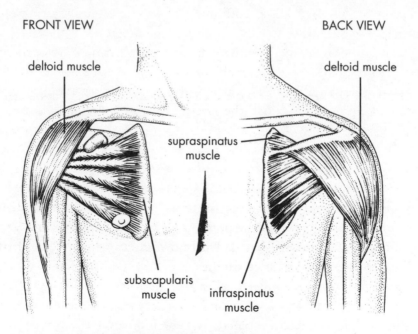

FRONT VIEW

BACK VIEW

deltoid muscle

deltoid muscle

supraspinatus
muscle

subscapularis
muscle

infraspinatus
muscle

FIGURE 4.2 Compared to the weight of the lever they have to lift (the arm) the muscles of the shoulder are seemingly dwarf to the task.

The rotator cuff muscles operate your shoulder's multi-directional hinge. They wrap around the head of the humerus in close, inter-weaving harmony, and by shortening as they contract, rather like puppet strings, they operate the long lever of the arm. As with so many things about the human body, this feat is remarkable. Your arm is extremely unwieldy in relation to the length and power of its controlling collar of muscles. All of them act at a significant mechanical disadvantage, which has important implications for the development of shoulder dysfunction.

The rotator cuff muscles lift and spin your arm in addition to their secondary role of hugging the humeral head to the socket to prevent it riding up as the arm lifts. The cuff also prevents your arm dropping downwards out of joint. Broadly speaking, shoulder problems stem either from stiffness at the pure shoulder joint, which is invariably coupled with poor scapula stabilising, or too much freedom of the shoulder joint, which leads to recurrent dislocation. Stiffness is more commonplace than looseness and may lead to over-use and inflammation of certain rotator cuff muscles or the eventual complete rigidity of frozen shoulder.

Competent rotator cuff activity naturally thwarts the development of our two main shoulder problems. Normal muscle action holds your arm down in the socket as it works and prevents the humeral head bumping up against the overhanging acromium, the bony ledge of the shoulder tip. A competent rotator cuff also prevents shoulder dislocation, where the knob at the top of the arm drops down off its socket.

Recurrent dislocation usually has a traumatic origin (most frequently during contact sports or falling on an outstretched arm) but shoulder stiffening to the point of freezing is insidious and you may not recall how it started. Dislocation, on the other hand, is dramatic and sudden as it catches the shoulder stabilisers (their protectors) off guard. Indeed, after the first dislocation, it is often only too apparent how silently and effortlessly the rotator cuff had hitherto kept everything in place.

As a mobile base for all arm movement, the scapula scoots all around the back of the chest wall. Thus the scapula provides a mobile stage of support; an invisible tier of mobility, even before your arm in the socket makes its contribution. You can demonstrate this for yourself: keep your arm fixed at the shoulder and simply manoeuvre your shoulder blade. Even without hinging your arm at your shoulder, there is a lot of useful movement at your hand.

The shoulder starts to lose power and performance when poor positionability of the head of the socket—caused by stiffness of the shoulder—combines with scapula muscle weakness, so that it cannot hold itself braced against the back of the chest wall to provide stable support for the arm. Simply using your arm badly—say, a hauling action by using the muscles of the side of your neck—can bring on both problems. Poor arm-lifting techniques involve raising your whole shoulder forequarter, as your neck shortens and the scapula wings out from the back of your chest. The hauling action abrades the soft tissues around your shoulder and causes them to fray.

Using the arm/shoulder properly involves automatically stabilising the base of the movement first. Even before arm lifting starts, the central core of your skeleton is braced by nipping in your tummy to stiffen the spine and anchor your shoulder blade When you lift a kettle, particularly a heavy one, you do this. As you lift you will feel the palpable effort of the body preparing a millisecond in advance—both the tummy reefed in and the scapula locking down. A good action deftly recruits the scapula stabilising muscles (lower trapezius and serratus anterior), making it easier to get a clean action of your arm working on its own at the ball and socket hinge.

By firmly stabilising the scapula as the base of the action, the small muscles of your rotator cuff suffer minimal strain because the ground does not move from under them. And by being placed in a better position to act, your neck muscles of the same side do not feel obliged to help. You will see in the section below that the hunching-lifting action of your shoulder is what leads to trouble—for both shoulder and neck.

WHAT ARE THE IMPORTANT ACCESSORY MOVEMENTS OF YOUR SHOULDER?

Like all joints and joint complexes, the presence of accessory motion is essential for streamlined performance. This is particularly true for your shoulder, which more than most needs everything going its way to work well. Here, accessory freedom not only gives the joint a youthful dexterity but provides vital internal manoeuvrability, which allows the proper lining up of the arm on the scapula for your muscles to work optimally. This critically enhances their slender margin of efficiency and directly influences power.

This is vitally important if you consider the unwieldy length of your arm and its slender muscle cover. Your arm is about 60 centimetres long and the muscles operating your shoulder are diminutive by comparison. This is quite unlike your leg, where the gluteals (particularly) are bulky enough to be grabbed in cupped hands. Your shoulders' rotator cuff muscles are slight and, except for the deltoid muscle, difficult to identify under the skin. They also work at awkward angles. When bending and straightening your knee, the hamstrings and quadriceps enjoy a significant mechanical advantage, both because of leverage (the angles they work at) and their ratio of power to length/weight of limb. By contrast, your arm muscles at the shoulder operate against all odds. Quite apart from their length of leverage, the spread from which they take origin from the bone makes it seem 'mission impossible' from the start.

When working against such natural odds, the positionability of the head, even by a millimetre or two, makes a difference. It is imperative there is minute but available latitude for the humeral head to manoeuvre on the rim of the socket. This essential freedom inside the capsule allows the ball to shuffle into position to get all your muscles (and their tendons) lined up for their optimal line of pull.

Accessory shoulder freedom provides just this internal manoeuvrability. Take the arm going over the head, for example. Ideally, there should be a small preparatory glide of the humeral head down on the socket, which puts the muscle prime movers in their best position to act. It subtly improves their angle of pull, which dramatically enhances strength. The arm floats up effortlessly above the head with never a thought.

All arm movements, major or minor, require this sort of preparatory positioning to facilitate their prime-movers. Without it, they are forced to labour at reduced efficiency with greater effort. Then, muscle strain is the most immediate, with stiffness and loss of elasticity the ultimate result. There are more specific manifestations, such as tendonitis caused by the friction of muscles working around corners and chafing against neighbours, which will be discussed later.

When the head rides up in the glenoid socket at the outset, these muscles find themselves in a shortened position and thus a slackened state; a point from which they find it difficult to contract adequately to lever your arm around. Like the villain in the movies who is forced to drop the knife by having his wrist forced under, if the muscles are put on the slack it is difficult for them to take up their length and achieve a powerful contraction. The gangster's fingers cannot close around the handle and he drops his knife.

Whether you use your arm to comb your hair, put your arm into a coat, or simply take a spoon to your lips, there must be sufficient accessory freedom of the head of the humerus to adopt any position it likes on the glenoid socket; each degree of freedom with its raison d'être to enhance its own dedicated action. Without it—subtle though that loss may be—the prime mover muscle labours to work.

HOW DOES THE SHOULDER GO WRONG?

Two distinct factors lead to shoulder joint dysfunction and, eventually, pain: poor stabilising of the scapula, plus tightness (and hence poor positionability) of the ball in the socket. In reality, poor control of the scapula is the most fundamental. In the first place, it is usually the result of low core stability and poor postural habits.

Using your arm badly involves poor stabilisation of the scapula through under-activity of the muscles serratus anterior and lower fibres of trapezius muscles. At the same time, there is over-activity of the upper trapezius—which span from the skull to the base of the neck and web out to the tip of the shoulder. When lifting (again, think of the kettle), the scapula fails to stay glued to the back of your chest wall but comes along too. It wings out from your back, like the buds of an angel's wings. This tangible defect of function is a very common misuse of the shoulder, especially with women, who are generally weaker than men. It puts the small muscles of the rotator cuff to greater effort but, just as importantly, by making the neck contribute, it causes chronic neck strain (*see* previous chapter).

Habitual misuse of your shoulder–arm complex is also a consequence of the very different nature of the scapula muscles versus the arm. The scapula muscles are postural and their mode of contraction a low intensity of long duration. They keep going during all the upright hours, maintaining the skeleton poised for activity. The rotator cuff muscles of the shoulder-proper are different. They are phasic; they only come into action when you want to do something specific, be it swatting a fly or conducting a symphony orchestra. They sweep into action with explosive effort to perform a specific task and then, job done, relax off-duty again.

When phasic muscles are weak the first stone is laid in the mosaic of dysfunction. When strenuous arm work is required, gross scapula movement is called in to compensate for lack of arm power. This causes domination of scapula activity over arm–shoulder function. Complications multiply at this point, through a primary tenet of neuro-physiology: overactivity of the postural group causes automatic inhibition of the phasic group. In simple language: as your upper arm becomes weak, its finer more articulate function is swamped by the clumsy gross actions of the scapula. The latter overrides the former. This unbalanced effort is known in clinical circles as reverse scapulo-humeral rhythm. Most of us demonstrate it to a subtle degree, though it can be hard to pick up by the untrained eye.

Beyond the natural disadvantages of the working shoulder, there is also the matter of habitual use. Most everyday arm work involves repeating the same few actions over and over. In addition to clumsy shoulder hunching when lifting, almost universally there is a lack of variety in what we do. Furthermore, most actions take place in inner range—that is with the area where the arms are pinned near the body (recall using a computer mouse, scraping paint, or turning a door handle) and we repeat these small movements ad nauseum.

Most actions are also inward pulling (bringing your hand to your mouth) as opposed to outward opening (throwing a frizbee or putting on a coat). This dominance of in actions, as opposed to out, creates inequity of strength and length of the muscles working your shoulder. As a result, you can become tethered one way and develop a degree of forward stoop of the upper back.

Predominance of one-way activity also closes down a component of accessory freedom at the glenoid socket. In particular, it squeezes the head of the humerus forward on the saucer-like socket, pinching it into closer contact at the front. The round bulk of the humeral head can be seen prominently though the skin, thus giving the shoulder a forward-hunched look, like the protuberant leading edge of an eagle's wing. Less obviously, it is harder to gap the ball away from the socket at the front, though this is usually unearthed only by deliberate joint examination. Both anomalies translate to difficulty taking the arms to full stretch backwards and up; the position adopted in a swallow-dive.

All these subtle anomalies set up your shoulder for trouble. Early on, simple dysfunction is not painful, just awkward. You become accustomed to having a weak arm, and unwittingly call in the scapula to help. By degrees, the dominant inward-pulling muscles contract down and permanently tighten, and the outward-opening ones become stretched and weak: the imbalance sets the stage for injury from trivial incidental mishap.

A chance awkward movement can demand urgent cooperation of muscles that are too mis-matched and discordant to respond with seamless ease. In that split-second when your arm should go out without skipping a beat, there is no fluent interchange of weak muscles taking control as the tighter ones let go. And without that flawless invisible mastery of coordination under the skin the joint is wrenched; an out-of-kilter system easily overwhelmed. As you reach over hastily to grab your briefcase from the back seat you feel a nasty twang in your upper arm as part of your rotator cuff is strained.

This is the first injury to a failing system. As your shoulder muscles clench in protective mode the joint loses its ability to ride out shock. Your shoulder becomes vulnerable to myriad everyday actions. When you least expect it you catch your handbag on a door handle and the pain is so bad you see stars. The limb that used to swing loosely at your side becomes an easy target to being annoyed. And this is how a shoulder problem snowballs.

Movement by movement becomes painful until, eventually, everything hurts. Even sleeping on the shoulder is painful. Automatic spasm of the muscles tries to guard against further unwanted yankings. One muscle in spasm introduces further discord and seeds more dysfunction, making additional shoulder muscles clench in protection. The problem becomes more widespread as each muscle in the plaited complex is injured and stiffens in turn. Eventually your shoulder cannot make any spontaneous movement without jarring. The domino effect ropes each in by turn and you eventually have a frozen shoulder: a general closing down of all-round accessory movement, which brings all purposeful function to a halt.

THE COMMON DISORDERS OF THE SHOULDER

Frozen shoulder

This most noteworthy affliction of the shoulder is where your joint progressively loses freedom and becomes painful and stiff to the point of rigidity. All movements become difficult but particularly getting on a coat, doing up a bra strap and combing your hair. In extreme cases, it is impossible to get your hand to your trouser pocket.

The problem usually starts insidiously, when the upper arm is achy and you suspect you have pulled a muscle. The arm may be vaguely sore beforehand and then you do something to hurt it, like pulling up the back-door button in the car when there is a momentary flash of pain. The agonising screech subsides with rubbing and soothing and you hope the hovering residual ache will pass. But in fact, your arm is never quite the same.

Although frozen shoulders vary in painfulness, advanced cases present a severely dysfunctional unit. There is virtually no movement at the shoulder hinge and arm action, such as it is, comes from heaving the scapula about. This is never more obvious than when attempting to raise your arm over your head, when your hand barely elevates to waist level and looks like a paralysed wing. To reach the door knob you must swing your entire upper body back. When lifting your arm out sideways from your body it goes only a few degrees before the scapula webs up and your hand flaps desperately down by your side. Pain and futile effort are the over-riding features.

Even in its incipient phase, frozen shoulder causes pain through the upper arm. It is often described as a deep gnawing in the upper third of the arm, which craves rubbing and squeezing. Unguarded movement is a curse, causing a sick-making wave of agony. Severe cases of frozen shoulder can be obstinately resistant to treatment, no matter what the course of action. One school of orthopaedic opinion says no amount of physical treatment helps and recovery will take two years, whatever you do.

There is no joint more susceptible to the right rate of introduced movement than a frozen shoulder. Too much action causes it to close down, as the cuff muscles heighten their hold, like a dog's jaws around a bone. The trick is to start off with small, unthreatening movements to eke out the first glimmers of joint opening. Gentle, rhythmic activity in the pain-free range provides the confidence to let go and start the juices running. If you are too exuberant and overrun the joint's ability to cope it will lock up again and set back recovery by days, if not months.

Severe debility is less common than grumbling lesser stages. Frozen shoulder proper usually restricts itself to those over the age of 55 but lesser grades are commonplace through all ages. On examination, your arm fails to move freely at your shoulder and the head of humerus is visibly bony at the front. There may be noticeable muscle wasting, with all accessory movements reduced. Gliding movements of your head backwards on the socket are springy and painfully resistant and your arm moves with reversed scapulo-humeral rhythm—meaning the scapula does more work than your arm. In less severe cases, this will not be obvious until the last degrees of elevation, with your arm beside the ear, when there will be a tight pain through the upper arm.

In least severe cases, the pain may be evident only at a point in range called the quadrant, approximately 30 degrees into the semi-circular journey down from above your head. A healthy floppy shoulder passes through this part of the arc by rising up and rolling over a hump but a bad arm will be stopped by painful restriction. This point maximally stretches the shoulder capsule (which shrinks at the front first) and is a warning the shoulder is losing play.

Supraspinatus tendonitis

Tendons join muscle to bone. Tendon tissue is silvery and strap-like with a mother-of-pearl sheen. Tendons have much poorer vascularity than muscles—hence their whitish colour compared to the blood red of muscle—and their limited lubrication means they are less equipped to cope with friction. Tendonitis is inflammation of a tendon.

Shoulder tendonitis occurs both when shrinkage of the capsule reduces the freedom of tendons to move and when the tendon itself shortens and loses elasticity. Friction caused by less room to slip-slide past one another causes chafing, particularly of tendons performing repetitive tasks.

Supraspinatus tendonitis is also the result of poor stabilising of the scapula. A hunched attitude of your upper back puts your arm in a poor work position, as the humeral head moves forward and up on its socket, bumping against the overlying ledge of bone. It also puts the supraspinatus muscle into a (shortened) slack state, making it hard to control the head. In addition, the puckering of the tendon makes it difficult to thread under the overhanging ledge as it tries to reef in its length.

Degeneration starts with a fraying of the tendon. In some cases a hole can be worn through the muscular cuff, which then exposes direct bony contact between the humeral head and the acromio-clavicular ledge. This is another source of pain. It is interesting to note that quite a high percentage of the ageing population has a hole worn through, or complete rupture of the supraspinatus tendon, with no apparent symptoms. Since the role of this muscle is more of a helper in lifting your arm—to bring about a better quality of movement by stopping your head riding up in the socket—your arm still works adequately enough without it. However, all the other muscles must work that much harder to compensate. Thus, the supraspinatus tendon becomes inflamed where it abrades under the bony ledge of the acromium.

With continual micro-trauma, a local hot spot develops as blood rushes to the trouble site. The damaged tendon then weeps, like a burn seeping clear fluid, and the exudate gets more viscid and sticky as it ages. Eventually the fluid becomes adhesions, which clag the tendon to its neighbours and gum up the works. The tendon chafes as it pulls past the other moving parts and a rasping inflammation is set up.

Freestyle swimmers are particularly prone to supraspinatus tendonitis—and it is directly related to swimming style. If swimmers throws their arms forward in a straight armed wind-milling action, assault to supraspinatus tendons is great. With each stroke, their arms ride up and forward under the bony hood of the acromium and abrade the tendons. If, by contrast, swimmers lift their arm out of the water as a short-armed lever, the elbows describing a careful arc through the air as their arm comes forward, the humeral head stays down and the tendons are saved. To do this you have to stiffen your upper back and stabilise the scapulae, giving your arms in the sockets room to move. Scapula stabilising also sets the socket in good position, with the round ball of the head to the outside tip of your shoulder.

WHAT CAN YOU DO ABOUT IT?

Correction of shoulder problems requires the loosening of the head-to-socket union and boosting scapula control. Simply speaking, this restores space to your joint so the head has room to manoeuvre. This in turn, helps separate the function of scapula and arm, to make them work more independently of each other and with the right ratio of input. At its simplest, the aim of treatment is to stretch the soft tissue structures that have become tight and re-educate a better scapulo-humeral rhythm.

More than any other musculo-skeletal problem, this is easier said than done. The pain-protection mechanism of your shoulders is keener than most and though stiff shoulders need movement, it is very easy to over-do it and make them worse.

Beginners

The elephant's trunk

If one of your shoulders has lost all function, this exercise helps restore the first glimmers of controlled movement. The pendular nature of the exercise makes it easier for your muscles to relax while slowly moving them into activity. At the outset, your rotator cuff muscles will flicker uncontrollably but persevering with these gentle, unchallenging rhythm movements for several minutes allows the muscles to slowly join in. As your muscle tone relaxes the tight capsule underneath is gently released by the movement.

The movement should be as unhurried and unthreatening as possible, otherwise you risk the muscles clenching and locking up en masse. The directions are for those with a problem in their left shoulder. If it is your right shoulder playing up, simply substitute right for left, and left for right below.

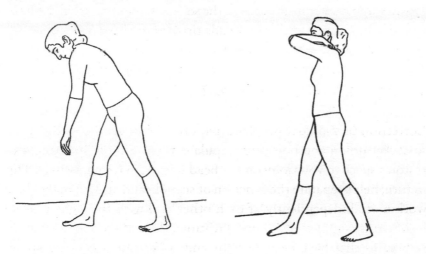

1   Take a step forward with your right leg and hold this stride position with your front knee slightly bent, your tummy held in firmly to control the midriff, and your left hand balanced on your left hip, allowing your left arm to hang by your side, its full weight gently pulling at the joint at the shoulder. Hold for a moment.

2   Swing the arm gently back and forth, increasing the magnitude of the swing as you can without jerking the arm, for 60 seconds, all the time keeping your abdomen braced.

3   Straighten your spine by pulling your tummy in hard and take your right hand behind your back and push your thumb into the tip of your left shoulder blade (scapula) to brace it.

4   With the scapula pressed firm, rest your left hand on your left shoulder and gently lift your elbow up and then down again. Repeat this short-arm lift once. Take care not to hunch your shoulder and shorten your neck here.

5   Release your arms and place your right hand on your hip again, adopting the same stride position as step 1.

6 Swing your right arm transversely, across your body, for 60 seconds then straighten up your trunk again.

7 Move into the short-arm position again, with thumb pressing scapula, and lift your elbow twice, keeping the shoulder blade firm.

8 Resume the stride stance and move your left arm in small clockwise, then anti-clockwise, circular movements for 60 seconds.

9 Adopt the short-arm lift position again and lift the elbow twice.

10 This series of exercises takes about 5 minutes.

Arm raising

This exercise is more difficult than it appears. The purpose is to stabilise your scapula, which is essential to lifting your arms. It also strengthens the muscles that lifting your arms up and back, to counterbalance all the lifting we do using the front muscles. Poor scapula stability often goes hand in glove with poor abdominal control so doing this exercise properly requires nipping in the tummy tight. It is important not to strain your neck as well, so take care to keep it long, doing the action as a clean ball-and-socket movement at the tip of your shoulder.

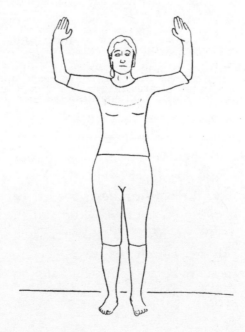

1   Stand upright with your back pressed firmly against a wall and your feet 5 centimetres apart.
2   Raise your arms out to your side to shoulder level, parallel to the floor, then bend your elbows up 90 degrees.
3   Brace your stomach muscles and press the back of your head, elbows and back of your hands hard against the wall. Your scapulae should feel like they are working hard to move together. This position stabilises the base of shoulder movement.
4   Slowly raise both arms just a few degrees higher and lower them again to where they were. The distance travelled is small but significant. Repeat this four times.

Intermediate

The shoulder hang

This exercise frees the tightness between your upper arm and scapula that develops through hunching your shoulder when you lift anything. It primarily stretches the muscles at the back of the armpit, giving you more length to raise your arm above your head while your scapula remains behind, pinned to the back of your chest wall, where it should be. While doing this exercise, try to avoid the temptation of letting your elbows bend as you hang. If your shoulders are too tight (and you have difficulty getting into position) you will need a lower surface, such as a stool, to start out on. You can build your way up to chair height.

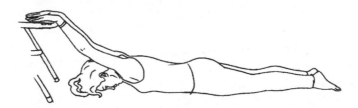

1   Lie face down on the floor with a chair about 20 centimetres beyond your head.

2 Lift one arm at a time and place the flat of your hand on the seat of the chair. You may have to push the chair further away if you find the front edge is digging into your forearms.
3 Straighten both arms at the elbows and drop your head through your shoulders to the floor. You will feel the pull diagonally up under your chest to the back of your armpits. Hang there for at least 60 seconds, longer if you can.
4 Slowly raise your head and lower your arms off the chair, one at a time. Rest for a while before repeating twice more.

The backwards shoulder stretch

This exercise primarily stretches the front of your shoulders. Opening your arms in this way pulls the head off the socket at the front, giving your shoulders more room to manoeuvre inside the capsule. You may encounter much greater restriction with this exercise than the previous one, though both are taxing. You will need a kitchen chair for this exercise but if your shoulders are too tight (or you have difficulty getting into position) you can use a lower surface, such as a stool. Alternatively, you may find it easier at first to sit on a pillow as this will lower the relative height of the chair.

1 Sit on the floor with your legs stretched out in front and a chair about 20 centimetres behind you.
2 Take one arm under and backwards (not over your head) and place it on the chair seat behind you.
3 Bring your other arm back to the chair seat and interlace your fingers.
4 Try to bring make your palms touch as you clasp your hands together.
5 Straighten both arms at the elbow and also straighten your spine as you thrust your chest forward between your arms.
6 Hold this position for 60 seconds then relax. Repeat twice more.

The reverse praying shoulder stretch

This is a complex shoulder stretch that targets both the rotator cuff at the shoulder and the tight union between your scapula and arm. You need to use a piece of furniture or structure with a flat surface at hip height—a broad windowsill is ideal—and it is important to get your back as flat as possible, with a straight line between the tips of your elbows and your hips.

1 Place your feet about 10 centimetres apart and bend your hips at right angles, leaning your elbows on the windowsill. Place your elbows just wide enough to allow your head to drop through.
2 From this position press your palms together, as if praying, above your head. Do not allow your spine to hump up but let your head hang down. Hold this position for 60 seconds.
3 To release, you will find it easier to disengage by bringing one leg forwards and bending at the knee.
4 With practice you will be able to progress this exercise further by dropping the hands, with palms still pressed together, onto your upper back. Hold this position for another 30 seconds and release.

The rolling-pin stretch

This exercise is a progression from the previous one, with the second part of it particularly effective at taking your arms to their natural limit of external rotation. Again, it stretches both the rotator cuff and the tight union between your scapulae and arms. You will need a kitchen chair and a rolling pin or umbrella for this.

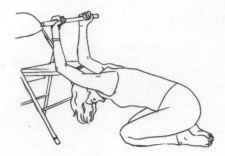

1   Kneel in front of the chair.
2   Holding the rolling pin with both hands, palms upwards, lean forward and rest your elbows on the seat, shoulder-width apart, then bend your elbows to 90 degrees.
3   Let your head drop down through your arms.
4   Hold this position for 2 minutes, breathing slowly and regularly all the time to help stay relaxed. This is a painful exercise and your muscles will want to tense up. Don't fight yourself: keep your eyes closed, your breathing rhythmic and let your head float away.
5   Progress the exercise by taking your hands further apart along the rolling pin.

Advanced

Lying-on-the-arms stretch

This exercise stretches tight shoulders—both capsule and muscles. Lying on the arms in this position stretches the plaited complex of the rotator cuff and also lengthens shrunken shoulder capsules as the head of humerus is levered off the rim of the glenoid socket. The shoulder of the arm closest to your body gains the greatest stretch. You will find that the humeral head of a tighter shoulder sits up proud and is loath to drop towards the floor.

1   Sit on the floor on a soft surface with your legs outstretched.
2   Bend both elbows at a right angle behind your back, each hand holding the other elbow.
3   Keep a firm grip then gently lie back on your arms, slowly lowering your head to the floor.

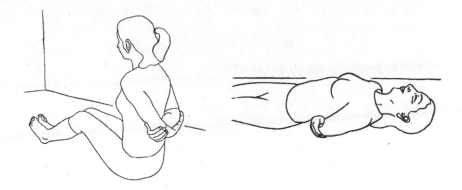

4 When in position, try to let the tips of your shoulders relax back to the floor, one cog at a time.
5 Alternate the cross of your arms so they take it in turns being closest to your back, deriving more pressure when your weight is on them.

The behind-your-back twist

This exercise takes the uppermost arm into maximal external rotation and the other into maximal internal rotation, each arm reinforcing the stretch of the other. It is a quick way of stretching both rotator cuffs from one extreme to the other, although if you have very stiff shoulders you will find it difficult to get your hands to meet behind your back. If they don't reach you can trail a strap from your top hand to the bottom one so your hands are linked. You will need a kitchen chair for this.

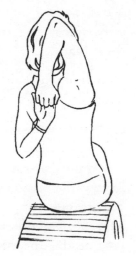

1 Sit on the chair and lift your right arm straight above your head.
2 Keeping your upper arm verti-cally upwards and as close to your ear as possible, bend your elbow and let your right hand flop down behind your right shoulder.

3 Turning your left arm inwards at the shoulder, take the left hand up high behind your back.

4 If you can, link your hands behind your back, keeping your right elbow pointing high up towards the ceiling. Hold for 30 seconds before releasing.

5 Repeat twice more then change sides and repeat three times on the other side.

The broomstick stretch

This exercise clears the shoulder joints right out. It demands the head of humerus roll right around the rim of the glenoid labrum with maximum laxity of both shoulder capsules. It also requires a committed contribution from all of the muscles of the rotator cuff to lift the arms—with control—up and over the head and down the other side. The important point is to keep the stick horizontal as it goes over your head. You must resist the temptation to allow one elbow to bend or one arm to lead the movement. You will need a long stick, perhaps a walking stick, for this. If you haven't got one you could use a broomstick or an umbrella.

1 Stand upright and grasp the stick with your hands about 80 centimetres apart, palms downwards. Begin with the stick held horizontally across the front of your thighs.

2 Lift the stick upwards, over your head then down behind your back so it rests on your bottom. Your fingertips will tend to pull away from the stick so keep a firm grip.

3 Reverse the movement to bring the stick up, over and back to its starting point.

4 Repeat several times in one generous sweeping movement.

5 Progress this exercise by bringing the hands in closer along the stick.

Handstands

This exercise is the ultimate for shoulder strengthening and infinitely preferable to using weights (15 seconds of handstands is equivalent to approximately 40 minutes of pumping iron). It recruits all the rotator cuff muscles to keep the humeral head from sliding off the glenoid socket and also demands maximum anchorage from scapula muscles to optimise arm strength. Handstands also strengthen the arms in an upwards—as opposed to downwards—direction. When you are able to lengthen your body skywards while you are up, you capture the superlative achievement of both strengthening and defying gravity from the opposite direction. Make sure there are no pieces of furniture nearby which you could strike if your first attempt fails and you come down sideways.

1 Choose an uncluttered space of wall and place your palms approximately 20 centimetres from the wall, hands flat on the floor, shoulder-width apart.

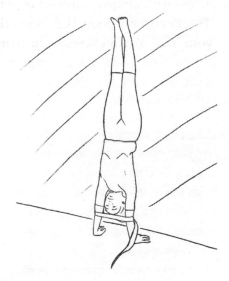

2 Bending both knees, inch in closer to the wall and then kick up with one leg first. You may need someone standing nearby to help you in the last stages of getting your legs up the wall.

3 Recruit extra strength by pulling your tummy in tight and jamming your shoulder blades to the back of your chest wall. If your arms feel weak you will benefit from tying a belt around both arms at elbow level.

4 Remain inverted for as long as possible. Initially this may only be a few seconds.

5 To come down, bend one knee and bring the foot to the floor as lightly as possible.

6 Repeat once.

Your elbows

WHAT IS YOUR ELBOW?

Your elbow bends the arm into two levers of manageable length. At first it might seem like a simple hinge but look more closely and you see it is not. There is a twisting subtlety in the working forearm that converts it from being a relatively clumsy robot-like lever—which, from a functional point of view, is pretty useless—into a remarkably graceful tool. The twist is brought about by two parallel bones in the forearm, each revolving around the other, carrying the hand along for the ride.

The ulna has a big role to play at the top end of the forearm, where it forms the main link with the humerus of the upper arm. By contrast, the radius plays the lead role at the bottom end, where it attaches to your hand. Your elbow is formed where the ulna links into the humerus, and the bony point at the back of your elbow, which you lean on, is the top end of the ulna. The front of the ulna forms a hook, shaped like a question mark. It makes a pincer-grip into a hole in the lower end of the humerus, so you can bend and straighten the entire arm halfway down its length without your arm falling out of joint.

The swivelling action of the lower arm is brought about by the two bones of the forearm dancing around one another, like two chopsticks, and this is the action that makes the forearm so different. The mobile chopstick is the radius, on the thumb side of the forearm, which revolves around the ulna, which is fixed to the humerus at the

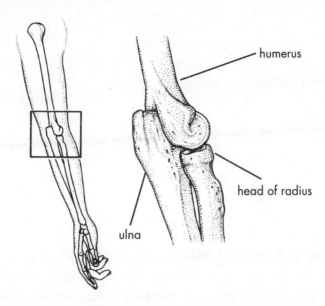

humerus

head of radius

ulna

FIGURE 5.1 The right elbow joint.

top end. Combined with a mobile wrist at the lower end of your forearm and your dexterous fingers and thumb, you can see what a devastatingly effective tool your upper limb is.

All arms exhibit a slight angle at the elbow so that when your arm hangs loosely at your side it harbours a slight residual bend. This noticeable kink gives the elbow a valuable tension, allowing you to carry heavy weights without pulling it out of joint. However, if there is a strong predominance of elbow-bending actions over elbow straightening, the elbow kink becomes more marked. You develop what is known as a flexion contracture of the elbow. You see this with over-strong weightlifters, whose arms hang bent at their sides like a gorilla. You will read below that this is just one of the ways your elbow can cause trouble.

HOW DOES YOUR ELBOW WORK?

The twirl and flourish of the hinging arm invests it with a peculiarly fluid motion, which makes it look living as opposed to synthesized. I'm often strangely discomforted by how humanoid robots can look.

I wonder if it is the element of an introduced twist to their append-ages—the perfect amalgam of several movements in one—that makes their actions so oddly real. By contrast, a doll's arm moves only up, down, across and back, with no hope of anything useful at the hand. The twist adds a third dimension to the movement. If you imagine a young girl plucking a daisy and bringing it up under her nose to smell you'll appreciate what I mean. This graceful action of her arm possesses—almost more than any other body movement—a delicate, streamlined, curling quality that makes it mesmerising to watch. You see it in spades when watching people practise Tai Chi. The movement of their forearms and hands is deliberate and slow enough to accentuate their spiralling quality.

At the outside of your elbow (with your palm facing upwards), there is a scooped-out surface at the top end of the radius that arti-culates loosely with a small bony knob on the bottom end of the humerus, which looks like the head of a pawn from the chess game. The head of the radius cuddles in snugly to the side of the ulna, just

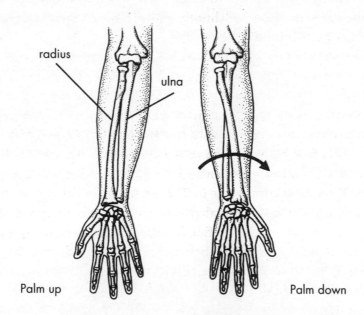

Palm up

Palm down

FIGURE 5.2 As the hand pronates, or turns the palm over, the radius swivels on its axis and the two bones cross. The ulna hinges with the humerus to bend the elbow.

below your elbow crease. It is held in place by a collar of ligament running around the neck of the radius and attaching back to the ulna. As the radius spins back and forth around the ulna, the hand— by being attached to the bottom—is flopped around too. You can demonstrate the radius bringing your hand back and forth by holding the crease of your elbow with your arm bent at a right angle. Turn your hand from palm-up to palm-down. When the hand is palm down, the radius lies crossed over the ulna, which remains fairly static. The main role of the ulna is to hook into the bottom end of the humerus to hinge the elbow.

Rotation in any part of the body is a crucial action as it allows us to address objects side on. This gives us better access to things by getting in closer, for example, bending down to pick up a carton from the floor, or contorting the forearm to play the violin. Rotation is particularly important to the human arm because so much uniquely human effort occurs at the fingertips and thumb. When threading a needle, you need to get right in there. Your arm must place your fingers exactly where they need to go. This skill, in combination with the bonus of your opposing thumb, makes for even greater effectiveness of your upper limb.

At its simplest, useful movement of your arm involves two specific actions: hinging the elbow plus swivelling the length of the forearm and cocking back the wrist. Take the movement of bringing a fork to your mouth, for example. What makes the movement so sensationally accurate, so you don't end up with tomato ketchup all over your face, is the ability to bend your arm to rotate the fork right around and direct it straight into your mouth—just watch a toddler trying to do it and you'll see how complex it is. The wrist action turns your hand around and at the same time aligns the thumb with your face. Once the stage is set, your fingers refine the hard-nosed elements of elbow and wrist activity and hone their accuracy with awesome finesse. Your hand crawls through space, tinkling the fingers with maximum purpose and minimum effort.

There is one problem in these precise actions: the repetitive nature of forearm activity, as seen over and over in different parts of the body. A deliberate arm action invariably starts off with the elbow straighter and the hand facing down, say when spearing your food with a fork.

Then as your elbow bends and your hand approaches your mouth, your forearm twists and turns your hand up to your face. To different degrees, this pattern of movement—flexion at the elbow combined with supination, or turning the forearm back—is repeated again and again throughout our daily lives, in countless different ways.

Cocking your wrist back is necessary for your fingers to work well. If you watch yourself pick up a telephone receiver for example, you see your wrist angling back so you can spread your hand wide in an open-stretched grasp to approach it from behind. This lets your fingers come forward and make their clutching swoop from the right distance. If you don't have wrist extension—such as you see with wrist drop paralysis caused by radial nerve palsy—you must lift the whole arm to drape the fingers of the flopped-down hand over the receiver so they can curl around it. It is a fundamentally awkward action.

Not surprisingly, supinating the forearm and cocking the wrist back is a much stronger movement pattern than pronating the forearm. While flexion/supination is repeated ad nauseum throughout your day, there is scant antidote activity, either strenuous—such as pushing your body up from the arm of a sofa—or light-fingered—depressing a piano key with the thumb. Furthermore, flexion/supination is a very strong action. This is why a workman's tools and household gadgets incorporate a screwing action (screwdrivers, can openers, door handles) that utilises supination over pronation. Incidentally, supination is strongest when the elbow is bent to 90 degrees, which explains why using a screwdriver is most effective when the arm is crooked.

The main muscle that bends your elbow is the biceps, the bulky Popeye muscle at the front of your upper arm. Simply speaking, it originates at the top of your arm and inserts into the radius just below your elbow crease. When it contracts and shortens, it bends your elbow. The triceps is its opposite number at the back of your arm, and it straightens your elbow out again. The important thing about biceps is that it always supinates the forearm as it bends your elbow.

The other main player in supinating the forearm is called the supinator. It and the biceps spin the radius lengthwise on its axis, carrying your hand from palm-down to palm-up. However, the movement incorporates a degree of compression of the outside compartment of your elbow as the muscles imperceptibly make the radial head slide up. This has important ramifications during overuse, as you shall see below.

The supinator muscle takes origin off the lateral epicondyle of the humerus, on the outside of the elbow (palm facing downwards), the lateral epicondyle forming the dome-shaped bulky mass on the outside of your forearm. You can see an impression of it through the skin of its fibres running diagonally inwards, just below your elbow crease. The fibres wrap around the neck of radius in a coiling fashion so that when they contract they spin the shaft of the radius outwards, bringing your hand around. This action unwinds the crossed bones (their attitude when your hand faces downwards) and it is brilliantly easy, which explains why supinator's action is so strong.

The muscles which cock your wrist back also start at the lateral epicondyle of the humerus, in what is known as the common extensor origin, or CEO. In contrast to the supinator, they travel diagonally from the outside of your upper arm, across the side of your elbow and down the full length of your forearm. They cross your wrist and insert into the back of your hand. As they contract (and shorten), they lift your hand backwards, thus cocking your wrist. It is noteworthy that both the supinator and the wrist extensors share the CEO. Thus, the site on the outside of the elbow is the single point of origin of muscles performing the two most common actions of your arm. In terms of elbow breakdown this is important.

WHAT ARE THE IMPORTANT ACCESSORY MOVEMENTS OF YOUR ELBOW?

There are two important accessory freedoms at your elbow: medial and lateral gapping of the hinge joint plus spin of the radial head. The first is best explained as the ability for your elbow joint to bend inwards and outwards at both sides of its hinge. Like all accessory movement, this medial and lateral gapping is a subtle hidden movement, not at all like the obvious bending and straightening actions governed by their dedicated biceps and triceps muscles.

Small dimensions of lateral elbow freedom make a tiny but valuable contribution to wrist action and thumb orientation. The extra dimension to arm/hand movement is not great—more like the bowing bend of a green stick. It simply gives your arm a workable compliance that makes small but critical alterations to the line of pull of the muscles working your hand—particularly the muscles that cock back your wrist, which we know to be a difficult action. In essence, a small inward deviation of your forearm at your elbow slightly lengthens the distance of the wrist extensors' span from the outside elbow to the back of the hand. It puts these muscles slightly on the stretch, which makes it easier for them to get strength of contraction to hold your hand back for your fingers to work.

Broadly speaking, the tighter the lateral compartment of your elbow (the outside when the palm is facing upwards), the harder it is to get these few vital degrees of inward angulation. In turn, this makes it harder for your wrist to cock back. Thus, excessive bending and supination of your forearm—creating an over-strong elbow—makes your arm develop a slight outward kink at your elbow. This throws the hinge of your elbow slightly out of alignment and also makes your wrist extension weaker.

Believe me, a degree or two makes a difference; the fixed angulation puts these muscles imperceptibly on the slack, unable to take in their length sufficiently to haul your wrist back. And here's the rub: if you cannot get your wrist back into extension, you have to compensate by supinating or turning back your entire forearm, particularly with sustained tasks like typing or using a computer mouse. This snowballs the problem. Strong supinator action laterally kinks your elbow more and thus the cycle escalates. Repetitive use of this combined group of muscles attached to bone at the common extensor origin can cause inflammation.

A freely spinning radial head is the other significant accessory freedom of your elbow. It allows the radius to revolve on its axis through its length so it can poise your hand anywhere in range between the palm-up and palm-down. Unfettered action all the way around contributes a vitally important background dimension to orienting your fingers and thumb and making your hand useful. This is critically important with finely calibrated precision work by your fingers.

As we see elsewhere in the skeleton, you often don't appreciate radial head freedom until you lose it. One of the earliest signs of this is poorer handwriting quality, so graphically charted by the written word across the page. Even minor sluggishness of radio-ulna freedom causes letter formation to become smaller and more jagged. The excessive strength of the supinator muscle may also make it awkward for you to get sufficient pronation to get the pen squarely on the paper. It can also be difficult cocking your wrist back, to keep moving your hand in advance of the letters as they travel right along the line.

HOW DO ELBOWS GO WRONG?

The two repetitive movement patterns of your arm are twisting your forearm back, thumb to face, and cocking your wrist back. You repeat these actions over and over again throughout your day. It is significant that two of the main players in these actions—the wrist extensors and supinator muscle—take their origin from the same piece of bone on the outside of your elbow, the common extensor origin (CEO).

As these muscles become more powerful from dominant use, their muscle tone rises. This is the natural pulling-in tension of the muscle fibres. Without simplifying the case too much, the stronger a muscle the greater its residual tone. Over time, raised tone leads to muscle shortening and this is evident in gymnasiums where body builders must stretch ad nauseum to prevent their joints crimping from their muscle strengthening programs.

The raised tone of the supinator and wrist extensors exerts a compressive effect on the lateral compartment of your elbow. Over time, this causes adaptive shortening of the soft tissues holding the joint together. In effect, the lateral side of the joint capsule shrinks and your muscles and tendons lose stretchability. This makes your arm kink laterally slightly at your elbow. The immediate consequence is twofold: poor angle of pull for the wrist extensors and less room for the radial head to move, each problem making the other worse. In addition, the try-harder muscle effort of the wrist extensors (in particular) exerts an upward pull along the line of the shaft of the radius.

This creates incremental displacement upwards of the radial head, making it bump up under the lateral condyle of the humerus, like the bow of a dinghy caught under a jetty. Over time, this impedes the swiveling freedom of the radius as the friction creates drag of the spinning radial head. Inertia must be overcome by more power from supinator to bring about the required movement, twisting your forearm back.

Thus the cycle escalates: your elbow kinks more, movement becomes more laboured and the residual level of tone of the muscles on the back of your forearm rises. As overactivity of wrist extensors and supinator becomes more obvious, the pinching of the lateral compartment of the elbow becomes more marked. In the same way that a door hinge only runs true if both sides open evenly, this lateral crimping makes your lower arm deviate outwards imperceptibly as your elbow straightens.

Opening in this skew-whiff manner means the rest of your arm must make adjustments to coordinate hand–eye function at the lower end. The compensations throughout your arm become so widespread that, eventually, even your shoulder has to twist inwards so your hand can work properly, and the strain starts to tell in your neck.

With tennis elbow the lateral compartment of your elbow is tightened. Occasionally, there might be a tight medial compartment, known as golfer's elbow. Your arm will gradually acquire trick movements to compensate for the loss of compliance at your elbow as your whole arm helps your hand fudge it. This eventually makes a simpler problem more complex; a domino effect making the local problem harder to unravel.

Elbow breakdown can be speeded up by using your arm for long periods with your elbow bent and wrist cocked. The mechanical disadvantage of the wrist extensors is further eroded as your bent elbow puts them more on the slack. Here again, your muscles have to contract harder to pull in their length to bring about the required backwards movement of your wrist. As you might imagine, this has important implications for people who use computers (particularly the mouse) or play the piano. You may be able to demonstrate to yourself how much easier it is to lift your wrist back when your elbow is out straight in front of you. However, with your elbow tucked into your side it isn't so easy. This is significant when this action is multiplied many times over, for the many numbers of hours people spend doing these things.

Over time, fatigue of the muscles of the back of your forearm causes the fibres to lose contractability and develop painful, cordy strands known as fibrositis. This condition makes your arm tight and painful in a dull sort of way and, more importantly, it lays the groundwork for wider spread, less reversible trouble of your elbow. Stubborn painful tightness of the back of your forearm lays the first stone in a gradually worsening scene. It also accounts for the commonly heard scenario of, 'I hardly did anything' to bring about a crippling pain that is difficult to move on from.

As the muscles on the back of your forearm become permanently shortened, the stage is set for acute injury, and this is where smouldering elbow problems leap to the fore. Low-grade inflammation of the osseo-tendinous junction, where the tendon joins the bone, is caused by micro-trauma of the tight muscle pulling at the bone. It moves into a different league when a stronger than usual jerk to your wrist (or forearm) causes the pre-tensioned tendon fibres to rip off the bone, simply because the muscles are too inelastic to go with the flow and ride out impact.

By nature, the elbow is very tight, as evident with traumatic fracture-dislocation of the joint. Without early intervention, the build-up of trapped blood can strangle the nerves and blood vessels within, simply because the pressure is so great. The sad result can be an unsightly and useless claw hand—a medical emergency that should never occur. Unfortunately, this natural tightness means your elbow has a diminished ability to ride out the normal jolts of everyday life. If you superimpose an additional band of tightness, in the form of a shrunken common supinator/extensor group, you can easily take the joint to the limits of its tolerance. In other words, it is easy to traumatise your elbow exactly where it is tightest.

As a final insult, almost as if it were a defect of creation, the attachments of both wrist extensors and supinator take place together over a tiny area. Instead of the common extensor origin being spread wide, to transmit the force of muscle to bone more gently and uniformly, it is localised entirely to the outer knob of your elbow where, even with healthy people, it often feels noticeably sensitive and tender just below the skin. Repetitive and forceful activity—either sustained wrist extension or repetitive supination of the forearm—zeros into this small area, creating low-grade inflammation even before tendon tissue starts being pulled off the bone. Even with un-athletic, non-tennis playing types (I suppose I mean computer nerds), sub-clinical inflammation of the common extensor origin is commonplace.

This problem snowballs once your muscles adopt defensive clenching in response to irritability and pain. This familiar guarding mechanism known as protective muscle spasm, is initially a product of inflammation, as we see so often in different parts of the musculo-skeletal system. It soon complicates the picture. Things rapidly get worse as the pathologically tight muscles develop fatigue from the build-up of lactic acid, and another element of pain overlays the previously tight muscles. The pain cycle ramps up.

THE COMMON DISORDERS OF THE ELBOW

Tennis elbow

It is one thing to use the arm in a sustained, low-intensity way over a keyboard, which invites muscle fatigue, but quite another to use both wrist and elbow together in a powerful slashing movement under load, as you do with the backhand shot of tennis. In truth, this is often the way it happens; a long-term low-grade lead-up with the outside elbow compartment slowly getting stiffer and less yielding, and then a sudden one-off wrench which is the last straw.

There is no action more vexatious to your forearm than the tennis backhand, although it is possible that other types of strenuous exertion (such as picking up a heavier-than-expected object with one hand, or using secateurs in the garden) can send your elbow into acute flare-up. Invariably, the tennis backhand strikes when your arm has become increasingly vulnerable; it bites more when your muscles are twanged tight like guitar strings. The combination of overuse and protective muscle spasm pre-tenses your muscles and the crunch comes when one big action tweaks them off the bone.

Shock waves are transmitted through the handle of the racquet into your clenched forearm, along to the point where the tendon glues to the bone. After the first tweak it is easier and easier to re-tweak it, with increasingly minor incidents. Each time you jar your arm there is additional microscopic bleeding as individual fibres ping off the bone. Blood and lymph accumulates between tendon and bone, which then organise into adhesions (or scar tissue) over time. Mending is made more difficult as scar tissue proliferates because it lacks an optimal blood supply and also lacks stretch. A small layer of scar tissue near your bone constitutes another interface from which your tendon can rip away.

Each painful wrench to your arm heightens the tension in the muscles on the back of your forearm. As they clench tighter, the threshold for what constitutes injury is lowered. There is a dull pain from the tight band of muscle running diagonally down the back of your forearm, which gradually becomes shriller as the condition worsens. Eventually, it is impossible to perform any useful task with your arm without invoking another painful tug at the outside of your elbow. Even picking up a teacup is painful (if not foolhardy) and it may be excruciating shaking hands or picking up a briefcase.

As your arm gets more laid up, you have the sense of wanting to pummel and knead the tight muscles with your other hand to make the muscles let go. You are acutely sensitive over the outer knob of your elbow and if you knock your arm—which you seem to do all the time—it is agony. Even people brushing past it in the street can make you defensively step aside.

What can you do about it?

Reducing the tone in your muscles on the back of your forearm is the first step in undoing the problem of tennis elbow. Without this simple first measure, pain begets awkward function which begets more pain and another cycle fuels in. You will see in the following regime that stretching both your wrist extensors and supinator muscles reduces their holding tone and makes them more accepting of shock. In turn, this brings about the first glimmer of opening of the tight lateral compartment of your joint, which is the ultimate vital clue to successful management of tennis elbow. Even the most meagre restoration of medial gapping of your elbow's lateral compartment restores a working compliance to your arm and creates a better line of pull for both wrist extensors and supinator muscles. Very importantly, it also does away with the need for both groups to overact and over-react, such an integral part of your elbow's declining spiral of function. It breaks the cycle of the ever-tightening lateral compartment and the tugging attachment of the common extensor origin and allows the irritable common extensor origin to have hours, then days, then weeks at a time without further assault.

As the hot spot calms down and the repair process continues uninterrupted there is a lessening of the protective muscle spasm. This in turn makes your whole forearm less touchy and reverses the cycle where your arm gets progressively tighter and more susceptible to the slightest jar or jolt. Loosening the union between your two forearm bones and restoring parity (in length and strength) of your flexors and extensors of both elbow and wrist is the next step. This makes your forearm more compliant and lets both sides of your elbow joint pull apart evenly to accommodate a wrench passing through. Improving all-round joint laxity and elasticity of your joint's soft tissues allows it to absorb trauma in the normal way joints do, like boats riding at anchor as a swell passes underneath.

In all but the severest cases, this is the best way to manage tennis elbow. Only as a last resort should you consider injecting steroids (such as cortisone) and/or local anaesthetic into the hot spot. Even though cortisone is often used, it alone will not rectify the mechanical cause. In the short-term it dampens inflammation and quells the pain. But long-term, if joint play is not restored in all directions, when the cortisone wears off the problem will resurface again sooner than later. With cases that are resistant to treatment, the best course of action is local cortisone concurrently with vigorous and sustained muscle and joint stretches. It is no use having the cortisone on its own. Incidentally, more than three cortisone injections is not advisable because it causes a weakening of your tendon fibres and a greater susceptibility for them to rupture.

Beginners

Pressing out the elbow kink

For this exercise you will push out your elbow with the heel of your hand. The pressure should be fairly hefty—enough to cause a strain down your outer arm—and you must move your pushing arm slightly to change the angle and find the sweetest pain. It stretches your outer joint capsule, gapping the lateral compartment and freeing the radial head from bumping up against the lateral epicondyle, which makes pronating and supinating the hand easier. It also stretches your very powerful supinator muscle, which can lose its stretchability through dominant use.

1 Rest your right hand on a low surface with your wrist extended and your fingers pointing back towards your right thigh.
2 With your right elbow as straight as possible, push the heel of your left hand into the prominent point on the inside of your elbow.
3 You can reinforce the strength of your left arm by tucking your left elbow into your waist and using your body to push.

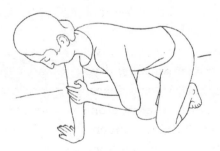

4 Keep changing direction slightly to find the tightest and most painful angle.
5 Gently lean into the pain, right to the point of intolerance and then withdraw, oscillating back and forth several times.
6 After you release your arm you may need to shake it to get rid of the residual discomfort.

Intermediate

The forearm stretch

This exercise is a complicated arm stretch for your shoulders, elbows and wrists. Overactivity of the finger and wrist flexors causes chronic tethering of the wrists and elbows, which keeps them short of reaching their full range. The first pose mainly stretches your flexor muscles down the inside of your forearms and then by turning your shoulders in by 180 degrees your forearms will go from maximum supination to maximum pronation. Both extremes free the radial head, though the second pose, which pulls the radial head down, will be an unfamiliar action for most and may require effort on your part to get the thumb sides of your hand flat on the floor.

1 Kneel on your hands and knees on the floor. Position your knees directly under your hips and your hands directly under your shoulders.
2 Turn both arms outwards at your shoulders, turning your fingers and pointing them back towards your knees.
3 With your elbows completely straight, rock gently back on your knees and feel the stretch running down your forearms and under your wrists. Hold for 15 seconds.

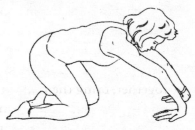

4 Gently rock forwards to your starting position, release your hands and turn them inwards, around the other way, so your fingers again point straight back towards your knees.
5 Keeping your elbows straight, and the thumb-side of your

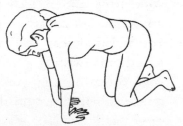

hands pressed down, rock gently back on your knees and hold this position for 15 seconds. You will feel the pull right down the arm.
6 Return to your starting position. Alternate with the arms turned in and out, doing each four times.

Advanced

The forearm twist

The main benefit of this exercise is to loosen the radial head from its tight ligamentous collar so the radius is free to swivel along its axis. Greater twisting freedom of the radius allows the two forearm bones to cross and uncross with more ease. As your arms are pulled out straight at the elbows your forearms are forced into greater supination, the upper arm more than the lower. This stretches the overtight union of the two bones along their length, which explains why the pain is felt right through your forearms to your wrists.

1 Sit comfortably in a chair with both arms extended straight out in front of you horizontally and your hands back to back.

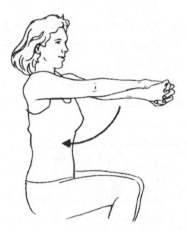

2 Bring your right hand over your left hand so the palms touch. Interlace your fingers right down to the web.

3 Keeping your hands locked together, bring them down and under, towards you, then up through the space between your arms and stretch your arms out horizontally again. You will find that this causes an extreme twisting stretch to your forearms and you will want to disengage your fingers. Try to hold your hands tight and straighten your elbows as far as possible. (Some may find their elbows remain bent.)

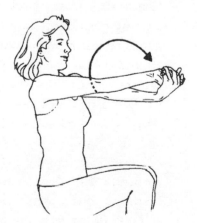

4 Hold for 30 seconds and then gently release.
5 Repeat three times.
6 Change sides, bringing your left hand over the right, and do the stretch four times.

Chapter six

Your wrists

WHAT IS YOUR WRIST?

Positioning and attitude of your wrist is important for optimal function of your fingers and thumb. You saw in the previous chapter how interplay between the radius and ulna directly affects the attitude of your hand. These two bones of the forearm provide large-scale background positioning, setting the stage for the finer movements further down your arm. As you get down to your finger-tips, precise function intensifies, with the fine adjustments of a hairbreadth superimposing themselves on the coarser ones, all the way back to the shoulder girdle and upper torso.

The shoulder blade (scapula) and ball and socket of the shoulder move your whole arm about; your elbow varies your hand's distance from your body; your forearm decides on the attitude of your hand but your wrist dictates the positioning of your thumb and fingers. By contrast, your lower leg has a minimal role to play in the function of your foot and toes because your leg is largely a pillar of support and ambulation, with very little variety in movements. It just keeps on walking. Your arm however, is called upon to provide a seemingly endless variety of actions, from the grandiose to the finicky.

The wrist proper is made up of the eight small carpal bones that act as mobile bases for your fingers. Simply speaking, they arrange themselves in two rows between the bottom end of the radius and the metacarpal bones of the palm of your hand. The metacarpals fan out from the front of the carpal block and join your fingers at the

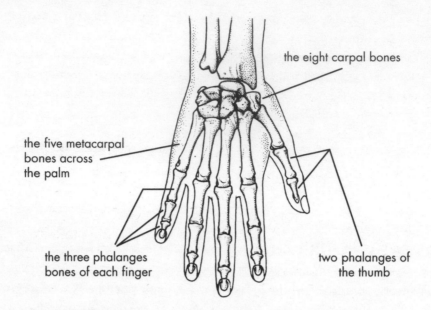

the eight carpal bones

the five metacarpal
bones across
the palm

the three phalanges
bones of each finger

two phalanges of
the thumb

FIGURE 6.1 The eight carpal bones give the wrist its circular freedom.

knuckles. They are fine slender bones that lie side by side, like bullets in an ammunition belt. Their ability to spread themselves out flat to open your fingers wide in a fan-shaped spread, or curl themselves into a tunnel to cup or mould your palm, is one of your hand's finest assets.

The carpal bones are situated at the base of your hand, just beyond the knob you see on the outside of your wrist. They spread across your hand in a 2-centimetre band, well down in the palm. The radius alone, on the thumb side of your forearm, articulates with the block of the carpal bones. By contrast, the ulna sits back, walled off from the carpal bones by a wedge of cartilage called the articular disc.

HOW DOES YOUR WRIST WORK?

At the bottom of your forearm, the sliding and gliding mass of carpal bones gives your wrist a cone-shaped 360-degree freedom, over and above the 180 degrees of forearm twist. As they take your fingers and thumb through range they alter the attitude of your hand's grasp. The carpi all squelch past one another as they enhance individual function of your fingers. They do this in the following way.

The eight carpal bones form two rows across your wrist, one behind the other. Roughly speaking they form up in two ranks, each serried pair dedicated to its own finger (though the thumb and index finger actually share three carpal bones between them). Take the little finger, for example. Back up in the base of your hand, two carpal bones line up one behind the other to contribute movement towards the metacarpal for that finger and thence on to the finger itself. This multiple, staggered source of fine movement gives your little finger a much greater depth of manoeuverability than it would have if it simply sprouted from the end of your palm.

These qualities are much more valuable to your thumb, since it is this appendage's genius quality of being opposable that differentiates us humans from our nearest living cousins, the apes. It is quite amazing how your thumb's metacarpal can rotate on its axis and roll across your palm, delivering its end to the tip of your little finger. This quality alone makes your hand profoundly useful, able to perform a seemingly endless array of activities, from removing a splinter to wielding an axe.

In truth, most of your thumb's generosity of movement comes from the junction at the base of the metacarpal with its carpal bone, rather than inter-carpal movement. But even so, inter-carpal play provides the vital ingredient that sets the stage for fingertip precision, as we shall see.

WHAT ARE THE ACCESSORY MOVEMENTS OF YOUR WRISTS?

Your wrist is actually one big bag of bones, jam-packed full of accessory movement. The movement between the carpal bones can best be described as synchronous. All of them shuffle and glide inside your hand, just like the tarsal bones of your foot, only more so. But there is one carpal bone whose movement is rather different. This is the lunate. This bone sits in the middle of the back row, right under the eave of the overhanging shelf of the radius. It is thinner at the back than the front—the palm side of your hand—thus giving it a wedge shape. As your hand moves and all the carpal bones ease up and down minutely, like finely honed pistons, the lunate goes along too, just like the others. Its wedge shape, however, makes it freer to glide one way than the other, which is significant in moments of duress for your wrist—particularly when it is forcibly bent back.

Mobility between the metacarpal bases is all important because it makes the palm mouldable. As well as articulating with the bottom row of the carpal bones, the metacarpal bases also articulate with one another as they lie side by side. As your hand is hollowed and the outside borders of your palm approach one another, the bases hinge open from one another, giving your palm a tunnel shape. The transverse pliability of the fan-shaped spray of metacarpals provides your hand with a cupping manoeuverability and thus a stupendous moulding grip for your palm.

Like all accessory movement, the freedom for the metacarpal bases is not great (there is much greater laxity between the metacarpal heads where the fingers join at the knuckles). But you will see later, when inter-carpal movement gets stiff, the metacarpal bases become almost rigid, as if the bullets in the ammunition belt have rusted. This means the metacarpals cannot ease away from one another to let your palm work properly and it affects both precision of your fingers and strength of your hand's grip.

HOW DOES THE WRIST GO WRONG?

Wrists suffer wear and tear when their work role is too heavy. Strong clenching and pulling activities, such as pulling on ropes, or jarring trauma from heavy duty tools can bring about wrist breakdown. Wrists also suffer when subjected to bearing weight, such as you see with walking on your hands, using curl-down handlebars on a bicycle, or strenuous pushing with your arms. Whatever the dynamics of trauma, the cause of breakdown is always the same: excessive squelching together of the carpal bones.

All eight carpal bones should ease and bob about beside one another, like ice cubes floating in a bag on water. En masse, movement of the block is like a symphony, with individual bones performing their small virtuoso. The movement of each bone is not great—but what *is* there is critical. More to the point, mobility *not* there is critical. If a single carpal bone cannot slip-slide past its neighbour it constitutes frank jamming of your wrist.

Repetitive strong, clenching, gripping of your fingers by the muscles of your forearm creates immense back-pressure through your wrist. The force of this compression traps both rows of carpal bones against one another, and then against the lower end of radius. Over time, the repeated on–off compression leaves the block of carpal bones bunched together and progressively less able to pull apart. All the bones are affected, making all-round mobility of your wrist below par, though no one movement is more painful than another. Strong clenching, with the additional jarring of a repetitive impact, is especially destructive for your wrists and this is why hammers, hoes, picks, axes and even hedge-clippers can cause wrist pain.

If the hand is forced backwards, the dynamics of injury are different to clenching. During wrist extension the capitate bone, which sits in front of the lunate, approaches the shelf of the radius. As it does so it squeezes the lunate out the front. The degree of wedging of the lunate varies from one person to the next but, broadly

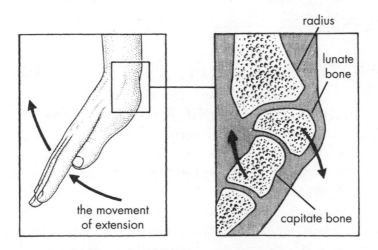

FIGURE 6.2 Forced extension can squeeze the lunate out of the palmar side of the wrist.

speaking, the more forcibly your wrist is pushed backwards, the more the lunate is oozed forward in the opposite direction, out the palmar side of your wrist.

Bearing weight through the hands involves both the compression of the carpal block and the squeezing out of lunate. Acrobats who walk on their hands are particularly susceptible to this cumulative compression, particularly if they overbalance and hyper-extend their wrists as they fall backwards. The most destructive forces on your wrists combine compression in extension plus a clenching grip with your fingers. This is why workmen's tools, such as jack-hammers and wood-planers, screwdrivers and saws, take a high toll on wrists, with carpenters high on the list of sufferers. There is great force through their wrist; cocked in extension with their fingers gripping the tool strongly.

Cyclists almost have a category of their own, particularly if they use downward-curling handlebars, which encourage weight bearing through their hands. Vibration from rough roads through the bike's frame adds to the toll, which explains the modern trend of racing cyclists crouching low (which also reduces wind resistance) and using forearm-support handlebars.

THE COMMON DISORDERS OF THE WRIST

The sprained wrist

A fall onto your outstretched hand may break the bones of your forearm, just above your wrist. This is called a Colles fracture and it is common to older women. The injury involves forcibly pushing the wrist back, which breaks the bone as well as sprains the wrist. To some degree, the bone breakage absorbs some of the impact and spares the carpal block from maximal jarring but, even so, the soft tissue insult can be considerable. Long after the bones have healed and the forearm cast has been removed your wrist can remain dysfunctional. There may be little outward sign of disability but your wrist may remain painful—especially when taking weight—and the grip weak.

The sprain is largely to do with squeezing compression of the carpus. The force squelches together all eight carpal bones and leaves them jammed, some more than others, depending on the force and direction of the injury. Palpating your wrist to assess mobility often shows the loss of a smooth contour of the bones sitting flush. Instead there is a higgledy-piggledy bumpiness caused by some bones sitting up proud and others recessed. Gliding pressure to the prominent troublemakers encounters a painful resistance, with a recurrence of familiar discomfort. Usually, the lunate is implicated at the centre of things, though it rarely dislocates completely (this is called avulsion) with rupture of the holding ligaments.

The most common wrist complaint is an earlier injury that never quite heals. The initial injury is usually a fall but it can be something more commonplace, like slamming a car door with the flat of your hand and your wrist angled back. We see a similar thing with using crutches. After a week or two the hands can be too painful to get about, simply because the wrists are not designed to distribute such forces. Hands are hands, not feet.

WHAT CAN YOU DO ABOUT IT?

Manual moving the carpal bones is usually a necessary adjunct to self-treatment. You can also achieve quite dramatic loosening of the composite carpal block simply by stretching the long finger flexor muscles of the forearm. These are on the inside of the forearms and the tendons span the front of the wrist and go through to curl the fingers.

Beginners

The interlaced finger stretch

This is a simple exercise that can be done countless times throughout the day. It counteracts the modern working posture by taking your arms high, stretching all the muscles that tighten when you sit for long periods with your arms pinned to your sides and elbows bent. It encourages the body to flow upwards, lengthening your neck and thorax in defiance of the weighing down forces of gravity that telescope your spine downwards. Of course, it also directly targets your tethered-in wrists.

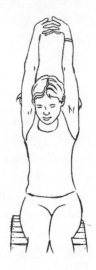

1 Sit squarely on a chair with your feet flat on the floor in front of you, your back held straight and your fingers firmly interlaced in your lap.
2 Raise your arms above your head, pushing your palms towards the ceiling while keeping your fingers interlaced. Straighten your elbows and ensure your upper arms are level with or behind your ears (from the side view your arms should make a continuous line with your body).
3 Hold this position for 1 minute. You will be surprised how difficult it is but don't hold your breath—breathe deeply and regularly as you do the pose. Your fingers will try to disengage but keep them locked tightly.
4 Bring your arms down gently, back to your lap. Repeat twice.
5 Disengage your fingers and re-clasp them in the next web along; repeat the exercise three times.

Intermediate

The kneeling rock

Since your thumbs and index fingers make such frequent contact in a pincer-grip action, the carpal bones on this side of your wrist are always tighter. Turning your hands out to lean on them makes this part of your hands bear weight, stretching the whole palm. The pressure causes the carpal bones to press past each other and greatly restores pliability on this side of your wrist and hand. It keeps your fingers and thumbs free to make precision contact (so long as your eyes hold out!).

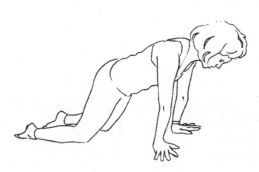

1 Start on your hands and knees on the floor, with your palms down and your fingers turned out to an angle of approximately 30 degrees.
2 Rock forwards on your knees so your weight comes over your hands and onto your wrists, especially the inner side of the wrists.
3 Rock backwards and forwards, each time attempting to go a little further forwards, for 30 seconds.

Advanced

The prayer

This exercise stretches your shoulders as well as your forearms, wrists and, most importantly, your fingers. The rotator cuff muscles of your shoulder often develop weakness in some directions and adaptive shortening, which makes for poor wrist freedom. This will stretch your fingers but it is important to keep all the finger tips opposed behind your back.

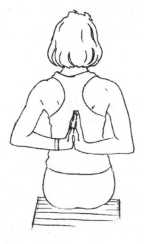

1 Take your left hand and then your right hand behind your back, bringing the tips of your fingers together and then the rest of your hands to a prayer position.
2 Press the heels of your hands firmly together and pull your shoulders back and down. If you have a stiff arm, do not allow it to hunch forward. Coax it into place.
3 Hold this position for 60 seconds then release.
4 Repeat once.

Chapter seven
Your hips

WHAT IS YOUR HIP JOINT?

Your hip joints are the ball and socket articulations between the tops of your legs and the bottom of your torso. Each joint consists of a round tennis-ball-shaped head of the thigh bone (femur), which fits into a deeply set socket (acetabulum) on either side of your pelvis. This articulation makes a modestly generous universal joint. It is interesting to note that as you stand upright, the cup of the acetabulum incompletely covers the head of femur, whereas if we kneel on all fours the coverage is more complete. This lends credence to the theory that we are descendants of creatures who crawled rather than walked upright.

The head of the femur is covered with thick, spongy cartilage with an opalescent, glistening surface to absorb shock and aid friction-free contact of the ball in the socket. The cartilage is thickest both on the top of the femoral head and the highest point in the ceiling of the acetabulum, where your full body weight bears down. The cartilage of your hip joints is critical to their health. The head of femur is kept in place by a sleeve-like capsule, a strong tube of tissue that extends from the rim of the acetabulum to the base of the neck of the femur, wrapping the two component parts of the joint together. The capsule is reinforced on all sides by dense bands of tissue—called ligaments—that add extra stability to your joints.

The design of the neck of femur makes it easier for your leg to access the side of your pelvis to fit into the socket. The neck is like a flying buttress or diagonal strut across to your pelvis and it makes an

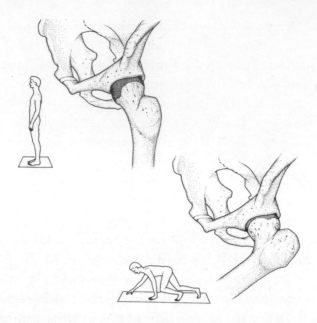

FIGURE 7.1 The cap of cartilage on the femoral head is most covered by the socket when we assume the crawling position. Top left: upright stance, left hip. Bottom right: crawling stance, left hip.

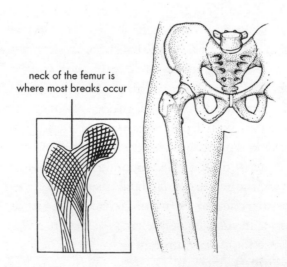

neck of the femur is
where most breaks occur

FIGURE 7.2 The hip joint. The internal struts of bone, or trabeculae, provide internal shoring to bolster the strength where the bone is most subject to stress.

angle of 125 degrees to the vertical of the femoral shaft. This is an ideal angle for re-directing your body weight through the shaft after it has come down through the femoral head. Internally, the neck of the femur contains multiple fine struts of bone—called trabeculae—which directly follow the lines of force through the upper end of femur. These bony filaments provide internal reinforcement where the bone is subject to greatest stress. Their confluence takes the form of tiny Gothic arches and the overall density of bone is much greater at their points of intersection. These points correspond exactly to where the bone needs the most help: the centre of the head of the femur, to withstand crushing; and the base of the neck of the femur to withstand shear. So here we have the beauty of nature repeating itself! Flying buttresses and Gothic arches not only in the finest cathedrals in the land but throughout our own splendid bones.

It is interesting to note that parts in the femoral head-neck-shaft arrangement do not have the benefit of this internal reinforcement, and these correspond exactly to where your hip is weakest and the bone most likely to break. A fractured neck of femur is common in the frailty of old age. It is rectified surgically by using a long titanium nail through the neck to prop the head and neck up again in correct weight-bearing alignment.

HOW DOES YOUR HIP WORK?

The main function of your hips is balanced standing and locomotion. Compared to your shoulder joints, your hips sacrifice mobility for stability. These joints are extremely strong and to a degree this is their nemesis. They are bound on all sides by powerful muscles to keep your torso poised upright on the femoral heads. The muscles of your inner thigh (adductors), outer thigh (abductors) and the glutei at the back fire off intermittent bursts of contraction, both to keep your pelvis balanced laterally and to prevent folding up at your hips. The gluteal muscles—by far the strongest—perform the most important role of propelling your body forward during walking. Even so, all the powerful muscles that work your hips generate upward forces to keep the femoral head rammed up hard into the socket.

The load-bearing forces sustained by the upper end of the femur are immense, with your body weight bearing down on a relatively small area on the crest of each head. These forces are intensified several-fold during the acts of running, jumping and hopping, making the maintenance of the femoral head a critical issue. A dense layer of joint cartilage is the first line of defence in protecting the femoral head, providing a resilient buffer zone to prevent the bone pulverising. Except at its base, at the osteo-cartilaginous interface, cartilage has virtually no blood supply and it is kept nourished by fluid forced through by weight bearing movement.

Cartilage is slow growing with a stately metabolic turnover. Synthesis of new cartilage is stimulated by on–off pressure changes through your joints within physiological range. New growth slowly forges up from below, like grass growing, as the top layers are worn off by movement. Thus, weight-bearing activity erodes cartilage but is also necessary for cartilage nutrition and health.

Each hip joint is encapsulated in a bag of lubricating synovial fluid. This fluid has three simple functions: pressure dispersal, lubrication and cleansing. Synovial fluid contained under pressure within the elastic bag of the capsule acts like an hydraulic sack or fluid dampener. Axial load is converted into outward pressure and works like a cushion of fluid to prevent grinding contact of bone. Optimum fluid quantity in your joints, plus the tissue tension of the hip capsule create a sense of walking on air, which absorbs jarring forces and makes movement streamlined. Too little fluid allows joints to clonk and the bones to chafe. Too much fluid makes the joints painful from the tension of the trapped fluid within the hip's capsule.

Synovial fluid is a superbly effective lubricating oil that facilitates glancing contact of the cartilage interfaces. Total immersion under pressure in synovial fluid keeps cartilage thoroughly awash and prevents drying and chipping. The fluid also contains large cartilage-eating cells—called macrophages—which devour floating cartilage fragments naturally rasped off during movement. The self-filtering process removes this gritty sawdust, thus preventing it lodging between the joints' surfaces and abrading the cartilage bed.

Synovial fluid is secreted by synovial membrane, which comprises the internal lining of the capsule. Secretion is stimulated by the fluid pressure within the joints, in addition to normal stretching–releasing of the joints' capsule. This allows the lubrication response to keep pace with demand when your joints are working hard, especially when subject to load. End of range movement is important. It prevents both capsular shrinkage and also stimulates secretion of synovial fluid to lubricate the surfaces. So, it is easy to see how full range weight-bearing movement keeps joints healthy. Another case of hard work being good for joints.

A balanced gait and even length of stride is an important factor in the health of your hip joints. Hips have a regimented pattern of movement as they angle back and forth during walking, and your length of stride is directly dependent on freedom of extension, the backward movement at your hips. Extension is the least generous hip movement and any loss will be more noticeable than a similar loss of the forward movement, flexion. The hip angles back only about 20 degrees but it flexes, thigh to chest, to approximately 130 degrees. Thus, a deficiency of 15 degrees in flexion will have fewer consequences than the same loss of extension, which is, well, almost everything.

WHAT ARE THE ACCESSORY MOVEMENTS OF YOUR HIPS?

Your hip is a deeply set ball and socket joint. Unlike its counterpart, your shoulder, it exhibits little shuffle and glide to provide laxity or joint play. Your hip is a sturdy, powerful joint and does not move with carefree abandon in any direction. Its most important accessory freedom is distraction, where the ball of the femoral head withdraws, or moves out of its socket in your pelvis.

On-off compression through the hip joints is critically important, both for nutrition of existing joint cartilage and synthesis of new cartilage. Healthy cartilage has the unwilling compliance of dense plastic, which dints inwards under compression and then springs back when the pressure comes off. This induces a suction–squirt effect to drag nutritional fluid up from the basal layers of cartilage, from the blood reservoirs in surrounding bone, with the greatest fluid shift immediately following joint loading and unloading. Fluid circulation through cartilage is heightened if the soft tissues are loose and stretchy enough for the surfaces to pull apart.

The manufacture of cartilage cells is stimulated by normal gravitational stresses through your joints, through normal extremes in on–off pressure. Thus, movement stirs the pot and stimulates cartilage growth, and this is critically important for hips, which suffer immense jarring from the impact of heel strike. General wide-ranging movement makes joint cartilage thicker and more elastically robust. Conversely, sustained high or low pressures retard the synthesis of joint cartilage.

Enforced inactivity, using a walking stick, periods of static standing, or simple obesity and slothful movement can usher in breakdown by depressing cartilage activity. Slowly, the cartilage becomes thinner and more brittle, which escalates as jarring forces are less readily absorbed. Hard pavements, marble floors and unsympathetic heel construction on shoes intensify the forces of destruction.

It may be counterproductive to rest a hip joint when it is painful. Although rest allows respite from pain, it fails to nourish cartilage and stimulate cartilage re-growth. Inactivity reduces circulation of fluid through cartilage and allows the capsule to shrink, thus physically limiting future movement and letting the grinding cycle take over. Although movement must be gauged by what your joints can take, arthritic joints get worse whenever movement is restricted.

Rhythmic walking with generous, even steps helps keep hip joints healthy. As you walk, a harmonious pumping action is set up, which greatly enhances blood flow through your joints. Alternating weight from leg to leg attenuates the blood vessels of the swing-through leg as the head of femur drags out of its socket. As weight comes on the leg again, elastic recoil of the stretched tissues slides the head back up into the socket. This is particularly important to the hip, where the head of femur has a notoriously poor blood supply.

Hip movement providing a mechanical pump also bolsters the role of a small but vital artery that feeds into the femoral head via the ligamentum teres. This short stout ligament attaches directly from the cup of the acetabulum to the top of the femoral head. When subject to hip distraction, its rhythmic attenuation and recoil shunts larger quantities of blood through to the head, like squeezing milk from a cow's teat, and a generous life line is urged through.

Walking also helps temper the bone of the femoral head and neck by the waxing and waning of natural gravitational forces. Stresses through bone prevent it de-mineralising and becoming brittle. On the other hand, eliminating gravitational forces—particularly with the weight-lessness of space travel—makes bone lose calcium and become fragile. In a more everyday sense, prolonged periods of bed rest, or simply using a walking cane or crutches, can actually make your bone less elastic and compliant. As your bone becomes less yielding, the demands on the buffering cartilage intensifies and escalates your hip's decline.

HOW DO HIPS GO WRONG?

Typically urbanised Westerners use their hip joints without imagi-nation, restricting them to regimented movement patterns. Although walking is good for cartilage nutrition it fails to keep the joint capsules of your hips stretchy. Walking may also be good for heart/lung function and the clearing of your head but its downside is its limited range of motion. Walking takes the hips back and forth through a rigidly stereotyped pattern. And when you sit, you simply arrest your hips at the 90-degree fixed point in their habitual plane of movement and at the end of the day you lie down with your legs straight, a position rather like standing, but at least not weight-bearing. We routinely utilise little of the hip's scope of freedom. Every now and then we might take a giant step on to a chair to get the biscuit barrel from the top shelf, or step sideways on the pavement to avoid a puddle. But, particularly in later life, we rarely use our hips as, say, a child does. As I watch my dear little elfin boy climbing a tree, one of his knees is up under his chin and the toes of his other foot are straining to get push-off from a bough far below, almost out of reach. Now that's using your hips!

More than most joints, the hips benefit from positional variety and extremes. Legs akimbo and separated widely in a resting pose is a very effective way of keeping hips young. Oriental people, with their penchant for squatting and sitting cross-legged, have a low incidence of hip disease and surgical hip replacement. Other societies are not so well off. Limited range of movement makes the capsules lose compliance and close out movement. With less elasticity and room to move, the femoral heads become more intimately held fast in their sockets. All-round capsular shrinkage keeps the femoral heads hemmed in to a narrow track as they travel back and forth over the same strip of cartilage on the congruent joint interfaces.

It is particularly easy for us to clip the freedom of the least-free hip movement, extension, and this routinely occurs with a leg-length discrepancy. A longer leg makes itself shorter by adopting a slight bend at the hip and knee. This adjusts the pelvis and makes the eyes level so they can focus (and judge distance), but in time it becomes irreversible and a hip contracture develops. The functional consequence of a longer leg is imbalance in length of stride. With every step, your spine twists one way as your skeleton compensates for the inability of the longer leg to angle backwards at your hip. It also means that the length of stride taken on the shorter leg is shorter. This small discrepancy becomes significant when multiplied by the routine 8000 to 10 000 steps we take per day.

Incidental trauma in the form of jarring or wrenching can cause rapid breakdown of your hip. One of my patients recently got his gum-booted foot stuck in a bog and, in wrenching it free, he sensed a small popping feeling deep in his joint. His hip remained painful thereafter and degenerated so rapidly that he underwent total hip replacement within months. From the mechanics of the injury, he probably avulsed (pulled off) the attachment of ligamentum teres and thus obliterated a major component of the blood supply to the femoral head. I have seen similar things done by forcing cross-legged sitting in yoga! But hip injury is usually a much more low-key and workaday event.

You may injure your hip hauling your leg into the car as you crawl in behind the steering wheel, stepping into a pot-hole, falling awkwardly while skiing, or simply walking on jarring heels. Whatever the mishap, the ensuing alarm causes protective spasm of your muscles on all sides of the joint. The first consequence is a tightness of your hip flexors at the front, which immediately prevents your leg angling backwards into extension. Automatically, the slim margins of freedom are narrowed further and your leg acquires a limp.

Limping is disastrous for hips. In some ways it is the first step towards total hip replacement. Once entrenched, partially through habit, a limp is well nigh impossible to banish and the consequences can be very quickly destructive. With your muscles clenching to prevent full movement, the underlying hip capsule is quick to lose stretch and the joint closes down further. In no time, your transient loss of range becomes permanent. For this reason, when your hip feels sore, it is important to take deliberately regular steps, evening out your length of stride, to stop the habit dead in its tracks. Limps quickly become established, but if caught early are still reversible.

Women universally have less hip extension than men. This is brought about by a tightness of the ilio-femoral ligament that runs down across the front of their hip joint. This ligament is shorter in women than men and accounts for the typically feminine shorter, daintier gait, not (usually) seen in men.

THE COMMON DISORDERS OF THE HIP

Arthritis

Osteoarthritis is the commonest affliction of the hip. It can be described as premature ageing of the joint where ordinary wear and tear has been intensified by outside forces acting upon your hip. Hips may be predisposed to degenerative arthritis by subtle factors such as discrepancies of leg length, where asymmetry takes its toll over time, or the consequence of more flamboyant, one-off trauma, such as bone fracture. Here, faulty union may leave your bones in poor alignment, which disturbs the lines of force acting through your joint.

Freak dislocation of your hip joint, though not common, can leave a legacy of profound damage. The trauma and shake-up causes stretching and tearing of your hip's structures, including rupture of ligamentum teres, which leaves reduced vascularity of the femoral head and marked scarring and fibrosis of the soft tissues surrounding the joint. Scar-tissue proliferation also greatly limits the blood flow and future mobility of your joint.

Whatever the original trauma, when your hip has been injured there will be a legacy of dysfunction that goes on to fuel future breakdown. The hip's relatively poor blood supply, its limited range of movement and the sheer powerfulness of compressive forces generated by its own muscles—remember the glutei are the most powerful in the body—make it susceptible to self-destruction. The daily wear and tear on these joints is great.

Cartilage destruction and poor regeneration is the first stage of osteoarthritis of the hip. The cycle of protective muscle clench starts to rack up when the synovial lining becomes irritable and then walking too becomes painful. The rate of breakdown is then almost solely dictated by the degree of muscle clench. Arthritic hips reach a point when they suddenly get worse. The most likely reason is the co-contraction of the muscles surrounding the joint, as they all adopt guarding mode (spasm) and jam the femoral head into the socket. Your hip feels stiff and painful and loath to move, and eventually your joint starts sticking or juddering on movement.

An acute arthritic hip often gives a jab of pain when rising from a chair and it may be difficult to bear weight on your hip and move off. Apart from limping, it may be difficult getting down to put on your socks or tie your shoelaces. Pain usually starts as a tightness in your groin or the outside of your hip over the ball and socket joint. Groin pain can become a gnawing discomfort, referred in a band down the front of your thigh to your knee, and it is common to think your knee is the problem! Pain is usually made worse by walking, though is sometimes worse in bed at night.

In the early stages of osteoarthritis of the hip, X-rays and scans can be confusing, precisely because they show so little. As it worsens, the narrowing of the joint space becomes more noticeable, as the cartilage buffer on both sides (acetabulum and femoral head) wears down. Later in breakdown there will be visible outgrowths of bone at the margins of the joint (osteophytes), caused by irregular weight-bearing through your joint. The painless juddering can become painful clonking and skidding between the joint surfaces as your leg moves.

As cartilage is abraded off the femoral head it loses its round tennis-ball shape and becomes flattened and irregular, a great impediment to streamlined performance. The head flattening also causes shortening of the affected leg, which leads to the characteristic rolling sailor's gait.

Like all joints, your hip has an idiosyncratic pattern to its mode of deterioration. The first movement to become restricted is extension (backwards), the next abduction (out sideways), and inward rotation (turning the foot in). The typical osteoarthritic hip gait exhibits a lack of all these: the foot is turned out and that leg is in close to the other, sometimes crossing over in front of it, giving a scissor gait. Because this leg cannot angle back at the hip, the length of your stride on the good leg is shorter, with your whole body having to twist to compensate. If your leg has significantly shortened through flattening of the femoral head, it will be necessary to take weight through your toes only while standing and your gait will become grossly exaggerated by dropping down on the shorter leg.

With total hip replacement so commonplace (the most successful field of orthopaedic surgery), one rarely sees hips like this today. However, artificial hips have a limited life-span and it is better to prevent decline in the first place.

WHAT CAN YOU DO ABOUT IT?

By maintaining all avenues of nonfunctional movement your quality of everyday functional movement is enhanced. This means undertaking generous movement, movement and more movement; even if your hip is painful and reactive.

The clue is to keep up the variety and range and reduce the high-impact. The ideal is to keep your joints juicy and slack enough to sluice wave after wave of fresh cleansing blood through to guarantee maintenance. Your joints must be kept loose enough so the head of femur can move about freely. This allows the forces to be distributed more widely across a greater surface area and does not gouge a single track in the cartilage beds.

Early attention to stretching, especially if you want to keep going with high impact sports such as running and tennis, will thwart the development of arthritic hip disease. Even though hip replacements are the most often performed orthopaedic procedure, following a modest regime of these yoga stretches will defy the day.

Beginners

The buttock stretch

This stretch helps disable spasm of the super-strong gluteal muscles that can ram the head of femur hard into its socket, rubbing opposing cartilage surfaces bare. The pose also stretches a tight piriformis muscle, which may be an added source of irritation. Piriformis irritability can inflame the nearby sacro-iliac joint, further fuelling the general hubbub of pain in your hind quarter. Find a clear wall with some uncluttered space in front of it.

1 Lie on your back on the floor with your bottom far enough away from the wall so that when resting your left foot on the wall, both your hip and knee bend at 90 degrees.

2 Bring your right foot up and place the outside ankle on top of your left knee.

3 Apply gentle pressure with your right hand and push your right knee towards the

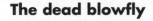

wall. Bounce it gently for 2 minutes, trying to push it a little further with each bounce.

4 Take your left foot down from the wall and change sides. Repeat once to each side. With practice, you will be able to add greater stretch by pointing the toe on the wall or bringing your bottom closer to the wall.

The dead blowfly

This exercise releases your groin if your thighs are pinched together by spasm of your adductors, particularly if your abductors are weak. The groin opening clears out the deeply-set ball and socket joints and creates much needed on–off compression over different territory on your femoral heads. Pumping both knees alternately by pulling them into your armpits allows you to get more range from each hip. If you have difficulty grasping hold of your feet you may need to loop a strap over each instep.

1   Lie on your back on the floor and bring your right knee up towards your right armpit, holding the outer part of your foot with your right hand.
2   Do the same with your left leg, so that both your knees and thighs are wide apart.
3   Bend your knees at a right-angle so the soles of your feet are parallel to (facing) the ceiling.
4   In this position, pump one knee then the other, alternately, deeper into each armpit.
5   Continue for 30 seconds and release.
6   Repeat twice.

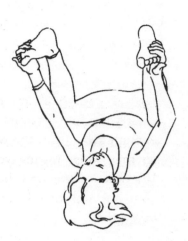

Intermediate

The up-and-down chair stretch

This exercise loosens your legs so your can walk more freely. It pushes one hip into extreme flexion while the other is fully extended. It stretches the back of the capsule of the up leg and the front of the capsule of the down leg. It also causes cartilage-stimulating compression on your femoral head. Because hip extension is a limited movement, the stretch is often felt more in the lower leg. The front of the hip of this leg often remains kinked, with a strong pulling sensation felt down the front of the thigh and your bottom sticking out.

1 Standing in front of a chair, grasp the back of it for stability and place your right foot on the chair's seat.

2 Sink down onto your left knee on the floor. If the stretch is too great place a folded towel under your left knee.

3 Keep your back straight and don't let your bottom poke out. If this is too difficult you may need to start with a lower chair or place a thicker mass under your knee (you could try a telephone directory).

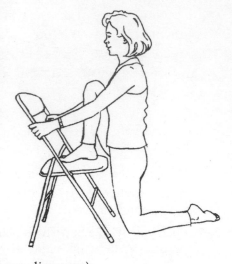

4 Hold the position for 30 seconds and release.

5 Repeat with the other leg, then once more for each leg.

Advanced

The knees-apart stretch

This is a very strenuous adductor stretch to help widen your base when walking, so you don't totter. Loosening your adductors also makes sitting much more comfortable, allowing your thighs an easier splayed attitude. The pose forcibly opens your groin through the weight of your lower body bearing down. You may feel sore over the pubic bone for a few days after starting the exercise, because this is where the adductors insert.

1 Kneel on your hands and knees with your big toes pressed together and push your knees as far apart as they will go.

2 Lower yourself forwards onto your hands, pivoting on your knees. You are aiming to place the front of your chest on the floor. Your bottom will remain perched up in the air and your feet will come up. The tighter your adductors, the higher your bottom will stay off the floor.

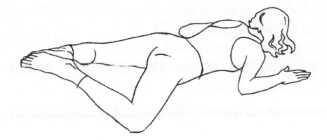

3 Remain there for one minute, breathing easily. Allow your knees to creep further apart as your hips release; this will lower your bottom.
4 Push yourself back with your hands and sit on your heels and rest.
5 Repeat twice.

The floor lunge

This exercise stretches the back of your hip capsule and makes it easier to cross your legs when sitting, particularly as you do when leaning forward to put a sock on. The more advanced version twists your hip into full external rotation. A stretch of this magnitude is necessary to coax elasticity from a very tough capsule, though the attenuating forces can be formidable and you must take it slowly.

1 Kneel on all fours on the floor and bring your right knee up towards your right hand.
2 Position your right foot in front of your left hip so that your foot rests in front of your groin as you straighten your left leg by moving backwards along the floor.
3 Sink your body down onto the right foot trapped under your left groin. Try to keep your body low and straight along the floor and resist the temptation to roll off the trapped leg.

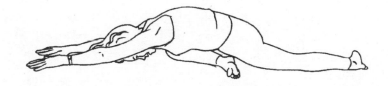

4 Maintain the position for 30 seconds and then lift your weight back with both hands.
5 Change sides and repeat once both sides.
6 Progress the exercise by moving the underneath foot in an arc away from the groin and lie down on it again. Maximum freedom of the hip allows your lower leg to lie transversely under your belly.

Chapter eight

Your knees

WHAT IS YOUR KNEE?

Your knee joint allows your leg to bend and, like your elbow, it resembles a simple hinge. The knee is formed by the union of the bottom of the thigh bone (femur) with the top of the shin bone (tibia). The smaller bone on the outer side of your lower leg (fibula) is not involved in your knee joint; it simply serves as bony attachment for muscles that work the ankle. The fibula does not bear weight. In fact, elephants are the only living creatures that bear weight through their fibulae. All the rest of us bear weight only through our tibiae in the lower leg.

Your legs fold up under you as you sit by bending at your knee, and both knees rhythmically bend and straighten during the swing-through phase of walking. This makes it easier to get your legs past one another and the momentum of the swinging leg helps to straighten your knee. Just before heel strike in walking, your knee is helped through the final few degrees by the large quadriceps muscles on the front of your thigh. They brace your leg back and then lock your knee, so you can bear weight with minimal effort, without the leg buckling underneath you.

The locking mechanism of your knee is an ingenious part of its function. The medial part of the quadriceps muscle (vastus medialis) helps guide the lower end of the femur in an inward swivelling twisting action as it locks your knee. Two crescent-shaped scoops of cartilage on the tibial plateau guide this locking process. These are known as the medial and lateral menisci and they endure immense wear in their role of locking and unlocking the knee.

The menisci are your knee's cartilages and they also help stabilise your knee as it works through range. As your knee bends and straightens and the wheels of the femoral condyles roll on the tibia; their passage is kept in check by the cartilages. Seen in cross-section these are pyramidal or wedge-shaped, and they pad out the gap between the round femoral condyles and the flatish surface of the tibia. Like railway tracks, the menisci dampen the potential wobble as the top bone rolls over the lower.

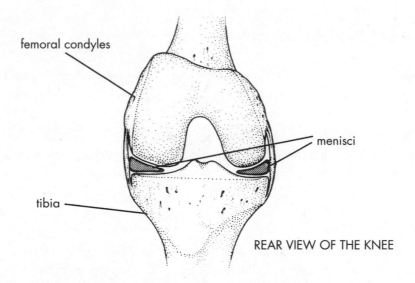

FIGURE 8.1 The wedge shape of the menisci pads out the space between the round femoral condyles and the flat tibial plateau.

The other mechanism involved in streamlining the function of your knee is the kneecap (patella). The patella is a shield covered in highly polished cartilage that floats in front of the knee hinge. It is embedded in the tendon of your quadriceps muscle, which runs from your thigh, across the front of your knee joint and attaches below to the tibial tubercle, otherwise known as the housemaid's knee bump at the top of the tibia. The patella is situated right on the bend of your knee and its purpose is to prevent fraying of the quadriceps tendon with its pulley action to and fro around the knee.

Knees commonly develop problems when bending and straightening fails to operate in the one plane. If your knee hinge is crooked —through your leg being bow-legged or knock-kneed—one side of your joint closes down and suffers greater wear. Just as importantly, your kneecap will not run true and this causes problems. As your knee bends and straightens, the patella fails to track properly as it glides up and down against the front of the femur. The friction created is a common cause of knee pain.

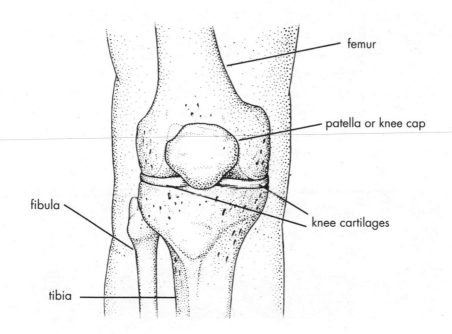

FIGURE 8.2 The right knee joint: the miraculous locking hinge.

There are two systems that contribute significantly to optimal performance of your knee—the menisci and the patellae. They suffer great wear and tear and are also the first to break down when your knee goes wrong. You will read below that patello-femoral and cartilage trouble are the two most common forms of knee trouble.

HOW DOES YOUR KNEE WORK?

The knee can bend from a straight leg to approximately 140 degrees, consequently your heel can touch your bottom. During walking it only bends through about 20 degrees. Knee bending is brought about by a combined rolling and gliding action of the femur on the tibia.

The bottom end of the femur is shaped into two rounded lumps called condyles, which resemble fat wheels. The femoral condyles fit snugly against two scooped saucers in the weight-bearing surface of the tibia, with the edges padded up by the menisci. As your knee bends, the condyles roll backwards over the surface of the tibia, while at the same time the tibia slides to the back of the condyles. This is an ingenious mechanism that not only means the wheel moves over the ground, the ground also moves under the wheel.

The movement of the tibia under the condyles ensures the femur does not drive off the back of the tibial plateau. With combined spin and glide, one bone moves in relation to the other, rather like the floor moving back under car wheels as they drive back. This feature of the rolling condyles does away with a yawning V-shaped divot that would otherwise open up at the front of your knee if it worked like a simple hinge. It also results in much greater range in the bend of your knee. As your leg straightens the opposite happens. The femur rolls forward across the surface of the tibia as the tibia also glides forward.

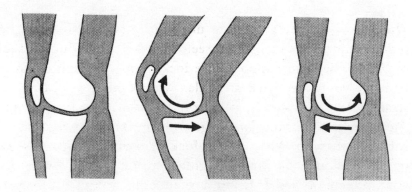

FIGURE 8.3 As we bend the knee, the femoral condyles roll back over the tibial plateau as the tibia itself glides back too. As we straighten, the condyles drive forwards, and the tibia glides forwards. Very efficient!

The condyles of the femur also play a role in locking your knee. The angle of pull of vastus medialis twists the femur in an inwards direction, which screws the two humps home in the two ring-shaped cartilages on the tibial plateau. As your leg approaches full straightening, there is an inward rotatory swivel of the femur on your lower leg, which snaps your leg straight. You can observe this when you look down as you brace your knee back. Without moving your foot on the floor you will see an inward swivelling clonk of your thigh as your knee pushes back through the last few degrees of straightening. This locking of your leg is performed by the femur twisting on the tibia.

The hidden femoral rotation makes your knee much more complicated than a simple hinge and it is vital to knee performance. Rotational accessory movement of your knee is even more critical than it is at other joints. A slacker joint like a shoulder, for example, can cope with a fairly significant loss of accessory freedom before dysfunction starts to show. This is because it has so many varieties of movements in its repertoire it can always find ways around deficiencies. In a tighter joint such as the knee—with its more singular purpose—that latitude does not exist. Even the slightest loss of joint play will handicap this very important function of your knee twisting to lock.

WHAT ARE THE ACCESSORY MOVEMENTS OF YOUR KNEE?

The knee's automatic locking mechanism is critical to its high performance. It overcomes the seemingly self-cancelling dual roles of bendability and support. The locking mechanism allows you to brace your knee back and relax when taking weight on your straight leg. Without it, you would consume vast amounts of energy simply keeping your legs from buckling under you. The subtle fluency of your knees locking and unlocking is even more spectacular during the highly complex art of walking. Each leg alternates between being a rigid pillar during the support phase, to unlocking easily and flowing forward to place your foot in front. Both knees deftly lock and unlock as your weight passes from leg to leg. No volitional control at all. Just sort of natural.

Forget about imagined miracles of walking on water. Plain walking is the miracle.

Your knee is a sensationally powerful yet subtle joint. For all its lissome compactness, it can take you from squatting to standing in one lithe movement. This feat alone is quite remarkable! It doesn't need counter-balances and locking pins; just its slender coating of muscles. The downside is that the locking mechanism is the first to deteriorate as your knee breaks down.

Less important, though still a factor with knees, is accessory lateral freedom of the joint. Like all accessory movements, lateral play of your knee is so slight as to be almost non-existent. A similar lateral freedom of your elbow imbues your arm with the sideways bowing bendability of a green stick, which makes it easier to achieve infinitely fine precision-work at your fingertips. The same subtle freedom helps at the sophisticated end of your lower leg's performance, particularly its adaptability to uneven ground.

The medial (inner side) compartment of your knee is freer to gap open than the lateral. The ligamentous shoring here is weaker—this also explain the predominance of medial ligament sprains over lateral. It also means that getting outward angulation of your lower leg is imperceptibly easier than inner. This slim element of lateral play provides the forgivingness for legs to stand sideways on sloping ground, and to also sit crossed-legged, knees akimbo on the floor.

When your knees start degenerating, their lateral pliability is the first to go and sitting cross legged like this is painful. In therapy, this is just the freedom we physios go after. We find that swivel and glide of the knees return more quickly when the lateral knee compartments are freed up first.

HOW DO KNEES GO WRONG?

Primary angulation problems between your upper and lower leg can cause degeneration of both knee joints and patello-femoral joints, as the poor alignment between femur and tibia throws into disarray the predominantly single-plane action of your knee. If your knee bows laterally, either in or outwards, a disproportionate load is borne by one side of your knee hinge. Either the medial or lateral compartment will be first to suffer wear. With bowed (bandy) legs, the line of pull of quadriceps moves inwards, which causes the patella to track diagonally sideways; in physics parlance the quadriceps tracking acquires a medial vector as your leg bends and straightens. If your leg is knock-kneed the converse happens; the patella drags diagonally to the outside of your knee as it bends and straightens.

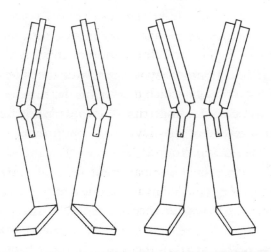

FIGURE 8.4 With bow legs (left) the kneecap tends to drag inwards instead of tracking true. With knock knees (right) it displaces laterally instead of tracking true, as the knee bends and straightens.

You can also develop primary patella problems if your knee does not straighten fully, although the mechanics are different. This is a common problem at the knee of a longer leg, where the slight permanent bend of the knee, adopted automatically to even up the sit of the pelvis, causes the front of the knee joint to nudge too closely in behind the patella and cause friction.

A lateral angulation problem of your knee can be alleviated quite simply by using a cork wedge under your heel. With a bandy leg, a three-millimetre cork wedge worn under the outside of your heel alters the alignment of the tibia under the femur and minutely changes the direction of the forces through your knee. Stress will be borne by a different part of the tibial plateau and the pain lessens as the cartilage regenerates under the heavily used area. The converse applies with knock knees. A small wedge worn under the inside of your heel makes the joint bear load through different territory on the cartilage bed.

Cork wedges mimic, in a much more subtle way, the old-fashioned orthopaedic procedure of wedge osteotomy, where a broad divot of bone was sawed out of the tibia and the leg allowed to mend again in straighter alignment. Think how much simpler it is to use a lowly cork insert! And effective almost immediately. Still, today, I find it nothing short of miraculous how just a few millimetres make such a difference, and my treatment repertoire would be lost without them.

Wearing one heel lower to make your kneecap float further out front of your knee may be useful in dealing with patella problems accrued from a fixed flexion contracture. Earth shoes have lower heels than soles, thus reducing the wear on both patellae. Deliberately lowering your heel pushes your leg more forcibly into a back-kneed position that disengages a too snug patello-femoral contact.

Secondary patella problems are almost more common than primary. They occur when your knee is affected by what is going on at other joints, namely the feet or the hips. Knees commonly develop patella-tracking problems when the inner arches of your feet flatten. This tends to happen as you get older and lose strength generally. As the inner arch descends, your knee moves medially (inwards), which alters the angle of pull of your quadriceps. In its early stages, this is dealt with easily by wearing orthotics in the shoes to activate your arches, though if the fallen arches have changed the angulation of your knees, medial wedging must be incorporated too.

Walking with your legs turned out like Charlie Chaplin, or turned in as with pigeon toes, also takes a toll on your knees. When your feet turn out at your hips, your foot operates diagonally on the ground. Rather than a direct heel to toe action, where your foot lands squarely on your heel and rolls along to push off with your big toe tip, it strikes the ground on the outer side of your heel then rolls the weight inwards over your foot to get propulsion with the inside border of your big toe. You will see in the following chapters how this flattens the inner (medial) arch of your foot and may cause bunions. The effect of inwards or outwards tibial torsion also means your lower leg is twisted at your knee when your leg swings through. This compromises patella tracking and may also affect your knee's ability to achieve lock.

Even small deficiencies in the relative rotations of femur on tibia can impair your knee's locking mechanism. Stability is the first casualty, in terms of lateral wobble, whenever your knee is bending or taking weight. The menisci of your knee become bruised and chipped; increasingly so the more your knee falls short of full straightening. Over time, this has a devastating wearing-out effect on the cartilages. Eventually, they are eroded away and bone rubs against bone.

If your knee is well aligned in the first place, it may be difficult to establish what makes your knee start to break down and eventually lose locking efficiency. The most likely reason is injury: minor or major. Even a minor strain will initially make your knee swell. Swelling is a complex issue because it is both the response to trauma and a source of irritation thereafter. When a good knee is wrenched the synovial lining of the capsule exudes fluid, rather like the mucosal lining of the nose streaming mucous if it is irritated. Unlike the nose, synovial fluid cannot get away and the fluid trapped in the bag of your knee's joint stretches and further irritates the synovial lining of the capsule. Thus, the swelling alone makes the joint uncomfortable, in addition to the original trauma.

Keeping an inflamed knee slightly bent makes it feel more comfortable because it depressurises the capsular bag and takes the tension off the synovial lining. A knee bent like this is said to have assumed its antalgic posture. In a matter of days, however, the slight bend may become irreversible, as the back of the capsule shrinks, and your knee develops what is known as a flexion contracture. At the same time, the inner part of your quadriceps (vastus medialis), which is responsible for the last few degrees of leg straightening, will develop disuse atrophy, making it doubly difficult to get your knee straight. Thus the problem snowballs.

THE COMMON DISORDERS OF THE KNEES

Irritation of the kneecap (chondromalacia patellae)

Chondromalacia patellae is inflammation of the underside of the patella and the front of the femur. It is the most common knee condition. In its healthy state, your kneecap floats well forward of the hinge joint, only occasionally making glancing contact with the moving bones, either when your leg is heavily loaded (getting up from a chair or walking down stairs or a steep slope), or when your knee is bunched in at a tight angle. Several sets of circumstances can thwart this healthy remoteness. The most general is a widespread general lack of looseness of your knee joint, the result of multiple loss of accessory movement.

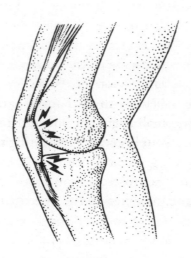

FIGURE 8.5 If the knee does not fully straighten, there is increased friction of the back of the kneecap against the front of the knee hinge.

If your knees are tight, the kneecap rides closer to the front of the hinge it is meant to be guarding. This sets up low-grade friction from the drag of the patella across the bending knee. Patella irritation is more intense with angulation discrepancies between upper and lower leg, when there is also a degree of tibial torsion, or where one leg is longer. Inequality of leg length is extremely common. The longer leg will automatically adopt a bent-knee stance to even out the lateral tilt of your pelvis. In time, as the bend becomes irreversible, the working hinge of your knee habitually abuts up behind the patella, too close for comfort, even when standing. The glancing friction can cause low-grade inflammation of the underside of your kneecap. This syndrome is commonly called movie-goer's knee, because the leg becomes much more uncomfortable during lengthy periods of sitting. It is painful to keep your knee bent and it is relieved only by stretching your leg out straight. Patello-femoral irritation intensifies with the addition of vibration, which explains why discomfort is worse when travelling.

With patello-femoral irritation, the cartilage of the underside of your kneecap is scored by close contact with the femur. Both the femur and the underside of the patella develop a furry surface that resembles a splintery board. The roughening causes patella drag as your knee bends and straightens, which adds to the general silting-up of your joint. The synovial membrane pours in extra fluid to sluice the surfaces clean and to dissolve fragments of cartilage, and the joint becomes visibly swollen. With the capsule of your knee stretched by the trapped fluid, the inflammation intensifies.

Low-grade irritation behind the patella is extremely common. Most of us have it to a small degree, although it usually takes hefty direct pressure down on your kneecap, while lifting the straight leg, to elicit pain. Sitting for long periods with your knees tucked in tight underneath and your legs crossed at your ankles can irritate the patellae by keeping them jammed in hard on the femoral condyles. This is a common position for computer users or people writing at a desk. With mild cases you may feel the knee audibly creaking as it bends and straightens, and you can palpate (and sometimes even hear) this yourself with your hand covering your knee.

When your knees are tight, the opposing congruent surfaces of patella and femur develop slight grooves, like shallow tram-tracks, to facilitate tracking. Sometimes the patella can jump out of its tracking grooves with turning or twisting movements, which is extremely painful. This is commonly described as the knee dislocating, which it is not. Though sub-clinical irritation has been brewing, a chance sideways movement with your knee slightly bent and loaded may bring you undone. The patella usually slots straight back into place, but the unwanted lateral movement further scratches the underside of the patella and makes the knee very painful and swollen. Whatever you were doing when caught off-guard, it is entirely possible to end up in a heap on the floor.

Acute lateral slip of a patella may be the beginning of a long history of knee trouble, especially if the structures holding your kneecap are stretched and weakened by the initial episode. Recurrent dislocation of the patella may require surgery to tighten the knee capsule or shorten aspects of the quadriceps tendon. In some cases, the tibial tubercle is transposed either medially or laterally, depending upon whether the knee has an inward or outward angulation. Moving the quadriceps insertion one way or the other alters the line of pull of the muscle and makes the patella track in a straight line as opposed to around a corner.

In severe cases of chondromalacia patellae, arthroscopic investigation reveals a mushy uneven surface on the femoral side of your kneecap, with long trails of seaweed-like tendrils hanging down underneath. Perpetual irritation and pain causes reflex inhibition of your quadriceps muscles, which affords relief by lessening the compression of the patella on femur. Over time, this results in marked wasting of the quadriceps of the front of your thigh. It becomes especially painful walking down steps, or down or a steep slope, since the muscles contracting as they pay out their length to lower the body results in much harsher compression of patella on femur. It may get to the point where even walking on flat ground is uncomfortable. There is a temptation to throw your leg forward from your hip and snap your knee back straight, to lessen quadriceps involvement in the locking process.

Surgical intervention takes the form of arthroscopic scraping of the underside of your kneecap to remove the mushy cartilage. I always prefer the simpler and less invasive approach: manually grinding the under-surface of the patella and then using another technique to polish it smooth. This sounds more hair raising than it is. Manual compression combined with small oscillations back and forth in the path of patella on femur polishes out excessive tracking groves and tidies up the opposing cartilage interfaces. Similar techniques are used in engineering circles, where flat metal surfaces are rubbed together to make them ultra-smooth. This is known as lapping and patients can use the same principles in self-treatment.

Initially, patella mobilising feels gritty, as if sugar is being ground between the cartilage interfaces, but within a minute or two the debris feels finer, like salt, as the grinding gets markedly less painful. After less than five minutes, the knee can be almost painless and the sediment inside can feel more like talc. This is another example where I am constantly reassured and gratified by simple techniques working wonders. After all these years I am thrilled over and over again that such simple intervention can make such a difference. Swinging your feet while sitting on a high table achieves light glancing contact of patella on femur that polishes the underside of your kneecap.

Torn or degenerated meniscus of the knee

If the screw-home mechanism fails to lock your knee it will show an imperceptible lateral wobble when it takes weight. The menisci are the first to take the brunt of this lateral movement, since their role is to wedge the wheel-like condyles into a specific tracking domain on the top surface of the tibia. They are sorely tried by condyles that constantly wobble and slew against their cartilage barriers when they are meant to run quiet and smooth.

When the femur is uncontrolled, the wedge-shaped menisci are exposed to the steamroller effect of the condyles rolling back and forth over the tibia and squelching against the cartilages. Trauma caused by the femur can cause the menisci to chip, split and tear, as bits of cartilage are torn free from the tibial plateau. Attrition can create a tag of cartilage with one end still attached, or a bucket-handle tear, which follows the circular line of the meniscus while remaining attached at both ends.

A fragment may be squeezed off the cartilage bed during a strenuous weight-bearing twisting manoeuvre when your knee is deeply bent. It then floats around inside the joint, sometimes getting caught in the hinge and making your knee lock painfully mid-way though range. When the fragment jams in the works it makes your knee give way when weight-bearing and resistant to straightening. If the fragment is still attached, the loose end can sometimes be floated neatly back into place by waggling the knee slightly, whereafter your leg will seem to function normally. It is unlikely the fragment will ever join up with the main bed, because cartilage has virtually no blood supply. It is possible, however, that the defective surface is eroded down in time through normal attrition, as old cartilage is replaced by new, growing up from below. Eventually the divot in the cartilage is sandpapered smooth by the normal wear of the interfaces against each other, and eventually your knee can become freely functional again.

If your knee goes on degenerating, the cartilage bed continues to erode and the joint develops slackness. The femoral condyles start tracking more loosely, bumping against the rails as your knee bends and straightens, eventually eroding the cartilage bed down to nothing—bone running on bone.

In the long lead-up to full rehabilitation, knees like this can be painful and swell after strenuous activity, even when there has been no wrenching incident. Once the synovial lining of the capsule has been inflamed it retains a lower threshold to irritation in future, particularly when your knee is taken to full bend. Problems multiply with the wasting of vastus medialis (of quadriceps) because your knee loses controlled locking.

Vastus medialis lies on the inner side of your thigh and can be seen as a soft mounded contour just above the inside of your knee. Its specific function is to take your knee through its last 15 degrees of straightening and screw-lock the femur home. In clinical practice one finds vastus medialis atrophied with all problem knees, no matter what the original trouble—patella or menisci. Your thigh is skinny and concave above your knee and the circumferential bulk is less.

Treatment in the past has often concentrated on restoring strength of vastus medialis rather than dealing with what caused it. Sportsmen would toil away for hours lifting sandbags to build up their quadriceps when sadly what they needed was restored accessory function. Walking with a bent knee keeps it weak, though once your knee can fully straighten, the strength of vastus medialis will return automatically. When your knee can lock back before taking weight, the strength of vastus medialis naturally gets involved. Conversely, labouring away to get vastus medialis strong when your knee cannot get straight is like hitting a man when he's down.

Operative procedures today for torn knee cartilages are a marked improvement on what they were. The realm of fibre optics has helped greatly in reducing the violation of knees. Arthroscopies are relatively non-invasive. Through a tiny incision, it is possible to insert a probe,

like a periscope, to view the state of the cartilages. If surgical intervention is needed, it is but a simple task to do it through the same tiny
incision. Gone are the days of the ten-centimetre scar and compression bandages from mid-shin to mid-thigh, followed by weeks of
rehabilitation to restore quadriceps strength.

Osteoarthritis of the knee

Your knee's menisci are its fibro-elastic buffer against the trauma of
bone on bone. They are your knee's natural cushioning and also its
locking mechanism. As such they are the first in line for preventing
destruction. If the cartilages are worn away, damage to the bony joint
is not far behind. Beware! This is the beginning of osteoarthritis; that
emotive term which conjures images of wheelchairs and surgical knee
replacements.

Osteoarthritis of the knee may be the culmination of years of
wear and tear, or the legacy of a major knee injury. Injury can tear
ligaments and/or break bone. Medial collateral and cruciate ligaments
disruption is the most common, and both cause long lasting
ill-effects.

If knee ligament remains stretched after an acute wrenching
episode, your knee will remain poorly controlled. And if a previous
fracture of either the long bones (femur or tibia) unites in poor alignment the bone will exhibit a minor angulation. This will cause altered
stresses through your knee joint and can expedite breakdown. The
consequences are more immediate if the fracture communicates with
the weight-bearing surfaces of femur or tibia, particularly if the
surface is not flush after the fracture unites.

If your knee's ligamentous restraint remains sloppy after injury,
the femur will wobble and knock on the tibial plateau and the menisci
will suffer in their buffering role. The medial ligament holds the
inside of your knee joint together and the cruciate ligaments prevent
shear of the femur backwards and forwards on the tibial plateau.

The cruciate ligaments are like a three-dimensional X that passes
from the bottom of the femur to the top of the tibia. One arm of the
X is taut when your knee is in flexion and the other in extension.
Slackness of the medial ligament allows the medial joint line to gap

open excessively and slackness of the cruciates allows the femur to shear excessively on the tibia.

Early on in arthritic breakdown, your knee goes through a dry, poorly lubricated stage. Starved of its own juices, the knee clicks and grates with extremes of movement, such as getting up from the haunches. It rarely swells and only feels discomfort after it has been in one position too long: either straight or too bunched up. In fact, these are the knees of most of us over the age of 35. Most of us stay at this stage but we can also intervene very effectively with yoga to make our knees 'younger'.

Normal stiff knees get worse if the capsule is allowed to remain tight. Like a woollen sleeve of a jumper that has shrunk in the wash, the capsule shrinks if it is not kept moving. If your knee fails to participate in normal romping movement it will lose play and close down. The capsule and its intimate lining of synovium become less elastic and easier to wrench during everyday movement. The damaged synovial membrane pours fluid into the joint and your knee will swell. This is the first step to breakdown.

As your knee's capsule tightens it holds the internal components more closely packed, which adds to the general friction inside the joint. The protective cartilage surfaces continue to wear down and their spongy buffering barriers get thinner and less compliant. Eventually, some areas can wear through to the bone. As a reaction, the bone becomes hyperaemic as it lays down more blood vessels and at same time, parts of the bone become denser (sclerotic) and look whiter on X-ray.

There is evidence to suggest that nerve endings also proliferate where the bone is subject to wear—in effect the nerve endings seek out the pain source. By this stage, your knee will be swollen, hot and painful and its range of movement limited. It will make audible scraping noises as the surfaces stick, then clonk past one another. Pain and swelling are usually the salient features with repeated acute flare-ups. Sleep tends to be interrupted because it is so difficult to find a comfortable position. Your knee may be very tender along the medial joint line and often needs the protective cushioning of a pillow to keep it aligned. Particularly in the side-lying position, this stops the inside of the joint gapping open towards the bed.

At its most acute, your knee may feel hot to the touch (indicating the degree of inflammation underneath) and tensely bloated with swelling. It will be locked in the vice of a permanent humming ache. As an acute flare-up subsides and becomes chronic it will lose its hotness and the swelling will become leathery. The knee itself becomes thicker and bending it is difficult, both from tightness of the surrounding soft tissues and the fluid trapped in the joint, like trying to fold over an overfilled hot-water bottle.

A chronically arthritic knee will not fully straighten and can barely bend to 90 degrees with a rock-solid end-of-range feel. The overlying skin develops a shiny, papery quality and the tissues underneath feel spongy as they emanate a smouldering heat. Movement is often associated with crackling and popping noises that can be likened to the squeaking of a rusty wheel. Elderly people may have to use a stick or a walking frame to get about, though knees degenerated to this degree are less common as knee replacements have come into vogue.

WHAT CAN YOU DO ABOUT IT?

Stretch is the answer. With the knee, as with any joint, a certain slackness promotes ongoing health. Looseness keeps it alive; the basic tenet of eternal joint youth. Joint laxity means your knee is less tightly bound, with more room for manoeuvre inside. The increased elastic give of the joint means the two bones are not so jammed together inside. The femoral condyles are less constrained into single trammelled tracks across the surface of the tibia, so they do not wear out a pathway as they roll back and forth. Equally important, the knee can get safely back into full lock so there is no wobble.

More than most joints, with the possible exception of ankles, knees can swell with the introduction of a new regime and this is often misconstrued as a sign to stop. It is important to get rid of the swelling because it can be a source of pain in itself, but it is just as important to keep going. Quite often a knee can be swollen and physically hot after these exercises and this is best dealt with by using ice. The best method is to rub an ice-cube over the knee, back and forth over the puffy areas which collect around the kneecap, until it has melted away.

My advice is to stay away from the surgeon's knife until absolutely necessary. Whatever is wrong, there are subtler, kinder ways of putting them right.

Beginners

Knee swings

This exercise is as easy as falling off a log. Relaxed, through-range swinging of your foot causes a light friction between the patella and the femoral gully. The glancing contact buffs off mushy irregularities in the cartilage surfaces, rather like sandpapering a splintery board. At the same time, the to-and-fro pumping action of your knee sluices greater quantities of synovial fluid through the joint, which thins the oil and vastly improves lubrication. Very importantly, the fuller tide of synovial fluid sieves out waves of cloudy detritus: super-fine cartilage fragments shaved off by the friction.

1 Sit on a high table with an uncluttered space underneath so that your feet can swing freely like a child perched on a swing.
2 Swing your knees, languidly bending and straightening with little effort.
3 Continue for as long as you like and repeat as often as you like—even a few minutes a day can help.

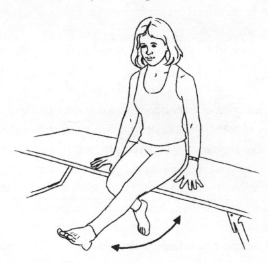

Walking on the knees

Walking on your knees is the most natural way of giving your knees new life. This exercise may feel counter intuitive because your knees may feel bony and sore, but usually it's exactly what they need. The forces through your knees press the patellae hard against the front of your femur bones, which subjects both cartilage surfaces to significant on off forces. This stimulates cartilage growth and usually—within days—your knees will feel as if they have developed more internal padding. The technique particularly strengthens your hip muscles, even more so when you walk backwards and sideways.

1 Choose an area of floor which has the thickest carpet and then add a folded blanket to make the surface as soft as possible. Using any nearby surface to help you, lower your weight down to your knees. Keep your back straight and your buttocks clenched tight so your bottom does not poke out the back.

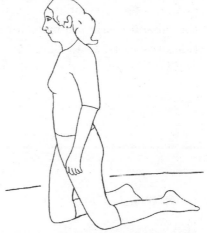

2 Take small steps on your knees, walking forwards, backwards and sideways in both directions for about 2 minutes per day.

Knee clenches

The specific role of this exercise is to capture strength lost by your vastus medialis muscle. This inner part of your quadriceps is responsible for taking your knee through the final few degrees of straightening. Vastus medialis usually develops atrophy from reflex inhibition when your patello-femoral joint is irritable, or when your knee cannot straighten fully because of physical blockage. In most cases, vastus medialis will resume activity of its own accord, once these inhibitors have been dealt with.

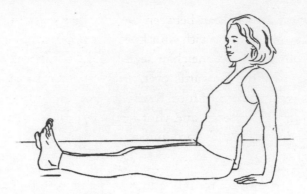

1   Sit on the floor with your legs outstretched in front and your hands resting on the floor behind for support.
2   Clench the thigh muscles of one leg first, then the other, attempting to raise your heels off the floor as you push back forcibly with your knees. Healthy knees let the heels clear the floor by about three centimetres but try to make each heel clear the floor by the same distance to keep your muscles in both legs balanced.
3   Hold the position of each knee alternately for 5 seconds, clenching so hard your thighs almost cramp.
4   Repeat four or five times with each leg.

Intermediate

The patella-grinding seesaw

This exercise stimulates cartilage regeneration through pressure changes and also sandpapers soft and mushy cartilage surfaces, making them smooth. Grinding back and forth seems unkind but it stimulates robust new growth from below. As your weight passes over each knee you automatically attempt to skirt around the painful spots as your patella presses into the front of your femur. You must forge on through and it quickly gets easier. Grinding should always be followed by the legs swinging to polish the surfaces and this combination is the best way of giving grunt to your knees. You will need two chairs for this exercise and and you may want a pillow on the floor to protect the knee.

1   Kneel on your left knee between the two chairs, resting your right foot flat on the floor with your knee at an obtuse angle in front.

2   With your hands on the chair seats, taking some weight through your arms, move forwards over your left knee so most of your weight is on your right foot. It will hurt as your full weight passes over your left kneecap and your left thigh muscles stretch when you are deep in the forward lunge.

3   Reverse the movement and then sit back on your left foot with your left knee fully bent.

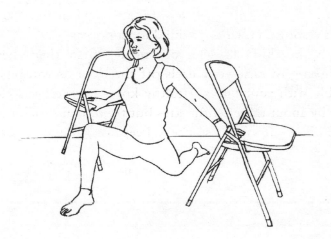

4   Continue moving back and forth for one minute. As time passes you will notice that the movement becomes less painful.

5   Reverse the position of your legs and repeat the sequence on the other kneecap.

A child's squat

This is an exercise people love to hate if they have bad knees. Even so, it is very valuable in a functional sense, simply because it helps you with squatting. People usually give up reaching down to the bottom cupboard as they grow older but you must learn to do it again if you are to bring your knees back to life. This pressure on the knees stimulates new cartilage growth and stretches the joint capsule, giving the patellae more room to move. The stretch also stimulates the capsule's synovial lining and prompts greater quantities of lubricating fluid to flush through when everything is running hot. Initially, your knees will go white with the strain and you will be counting the seconds until it is over.

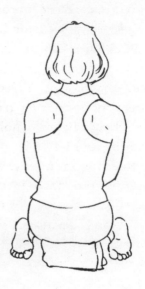

1 Kneel on the floor with your knees together and a small cushion between your ankles.
2 Widen the gap between your feet to about 30 centimetres, keeping the upper side of your feet on the floor and your toes pointing straight back.
3 Lower your bottom down on to the cushion, keeping your knees together as you do, and sit there for one minute. People with loose knees may not need the cushion; others with tighter knees may need several cushions.
4 Ease forwards and take the weight off your feet.

Advanced

The sitting bowl

This exercise restores torsion between your upper and lower leg, making it easier to achieve locking of your knee. The small inward rotation of the femur on the tibia to brace the leg is always the first accessory movement to be lost in this joint and frequently normal knees complain in this position. Invariably, one knee is tighter and the outer border of your foot will not lie down sideways on the carpet. This will be your problem knee and gentle pressure with your hand against your heel will be felt in the knee. The pressure of your bottom sitting on your heels increases the tibial torsion and you can accentu-ate this further by swivelling your bottom left and right to press the heels out further.

1   Kneel on the floor.
2   Press your big toes together, hook your thumbs around the inner side of your heels and pull them outwards.
3   With the heels widely sepa-rated and big toes together, lower your bottom down into the bowl-shaped hollow made by your feet.
4   Sit there for one minute with your bottom pressing your heels apart. During this time you can oscillate your bottom left and right to further force the heels apart.
5   Release and relax and repeat once more.

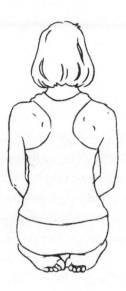

Chapter nine

Your ankles

WHAT IS YOUR ANKLE?

The ankle complex is an unusual one. It provides hinge movement during walking, so you can strike the ground with your heel and proceed through to push-off with your toes, while at the same time it provides lateral stability so you can balance on your foot on the ground. Strictly speaking, your ankle is a hinge that connects your lower leg with your foot. The two bones of your lower leg, the tibia (the larger on the inner side) and the fibula (the outside), make a mortice, which contains the uppermost bone of your foot, the talus. Several tarsal bones make up the mid-foot and these stack themselves around in an arch, with the talus perched on top.

The tibia bears weight with the top of the talus, whereas the fibula makes only glancing contact with the outer side, thus boxing the talus in. The fibula ends lower down the side of the talus than the tibia, and if you look at your own foot you will see your outer anklebone is lower and further back. At the start this is significant because it encourages your foot to turn under in the classical ankle-straining injury.

The upper weight-bearing surface of the talus is shaped like a dome. As you point your toe (plantarflex) the dome rolls out from under the bottom end of the tibia. As you bring your foot back towards you (dorsiflex) it rolls back under the eave again. You can palpate your foot doing this and almost feel the rounded protuberance of talus rolling out and back at the front of your ankle.

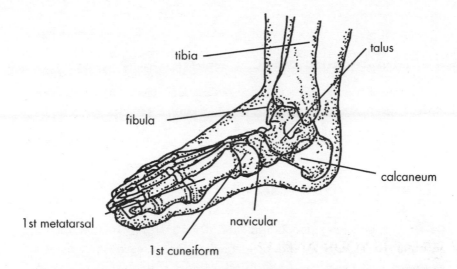

tibia

talus

fibula

calcaneum

1st metatarsal

navicular

1st cuneiform

FIGURE 9.1 The talus, at the top of the arch of the foot, sits locked in the jaws of the tibia and fibula coming down on them from above.

With the talus sitting at the top of the arch, the rest of your foot spans out below, like a sandstone arch of a Roman bridge. The talus does not sit quite squarely between the two anklebones; it has a slight inward attitude at the front as it makes contact with the rest of your foot below. This twisted orientation has important ramifications in malfunction of your foot, as we shall later see.

The talus makes a joint with the heel bone (calcaneum), which sits below it and further back, and also with the front of the foot through the navicular bone. Thus talus distributes stress both ways down through the arch: back through the calcaneum and forward through the navicular, tarsal bones and the five metatarsal bones. The meta-tarsals splay out across the front of your foot like a fan, from the front of the tarsal block. The loosely held parallel union of these five slender bones gives the forefoot fantastic lateral pliability. The toes attach to the front ends of the metatarsal (the heads) and provide your grabbing-the-ground forward propulsion plus extra foot stability.

The ideal forefoot bears weight primarily on the heads of the first and fifth metatarsal, where they join the big and little toes. The heel bears a little over half your body-weight and the forefoot shares the rest. Poorly functioning feet bear weight on all metatarsal heads, not just the outer two. The second metatarsal head in particular often develops a painful skin callus near the centre of the ball of your foot, the callus being build-up of soft tissue to help protect the bone. As it proliferates it can become painful to walk and needs paring back by a chiropodist. Your foot can also be made more painful by shoes that pinch the toes or have too high a heel.

HOW DOES YOUR ANKLE WORK?

Pure ankle movement is plantar- and dorsiflexion, which is pointing the toe and cocking the foot back. The inward and outward movement takes place at the sub-talar joint, as the bony arch of your foot slides medially and laterally under the talus. The amalgam of these movements allows your semi-rigid lower leg to balance on the ground. For the purposes of this chapter, the ankle and the sub-talar joints will be discussed together.

The design of the human foot is exquisitely beautiful; another masterpiece of engineering at its best. The squashing forces trans-mitted through the crest of your foot's bony arch are immense and several factors contribute in helping it disperse the load. In addition to the natural stacking of the mid-foot bones into an arch, tension of muscles and ligaments spanning the underside helps keep the vault of your foot high. As you will see in the next chapter, your toe muscles play a major role in keeping the bottom of the arch pinched together, like catgut stretched across a bow. However, the nearer one gets to the crest of the arch, the harder it is to dissipate the forces of compression. This is where the dynamics of the talus, the keystone of the arch, come in.

Two important muscles—tibialis anterior and tibialis posterior—share the role of actively hauling your foot's arch up. They have a curious action because neither works directly on the talus, the pediment at the top of the vault. Instead they target the bones imme-diately below in the arch, squeezing them together to pinch the talus skyward. This stops the talus falling through to the floor and the arch smashing flat.

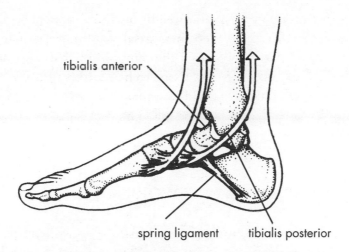

tibialis anterior

spring ligament   tibialis posterior

FIGURE 9.2 The spring ligament passes from the calcaneum to the navicular and keeps the talus pinched high.

Tibialis anterior is the long fleshy muscle just to the outside of your shin bone. It crosses to the top of your foot on the inside front of your ankle and attaches to the first cuneiform at the top of your forefoot, to navicular and the first metatarsal. It lifts the arch on the inside of your foot and you can see its tendon webbing up at the inner side of your ankle if you cock your toes back towards you, turning the underside of the foot up.

Tibialis posterior comes down from the back of the calf, hooks around the inside ankle bone and approaches navicular from the underside of your foot. It approaches this same bone from the opposite direction to the tibialis anterior and also pinches the sides of the arch together to keep the foot vault held high. You can identify this muscle by pointing your toes downwards and turning your foot in, as if inspecting the sole of your foot.

In summary, tibialis anterior hauls the top of the arch up from above, while tibialis posterior, by pulling the navicular bone down and back towards your heel, pinches the sides of the arch into a more acute peak. It is a brilliant mechanism! Two strong and dominant muscles sharing the role of preventing body weight flattening the foot's arch. One muscle works when the toe is pointed, and the other when the foot is cocked—each when the foot is turned in. The inner arch needs the double strength of both tibialis muscles holding it up because it is so directly involved in the dissipation of forces through your foot. If this arch collapses, the talus will screw down and your foot will lose its capacity to spring with push-off for each step.

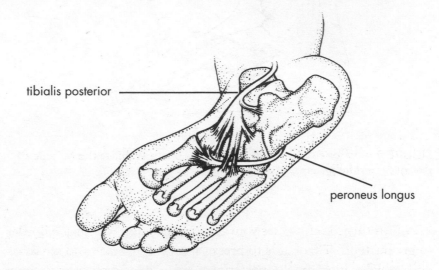

FIGURE 9.3 The cross-over of tibialis posterior and peroneus longus acts like an elastic stirrup suspending the ach of the foot and keeping the forefoot flat on the floor.

Peroneus longus balances the action of both tibialis posterior and anterior by lifting up the outside border of your foot. It swings around under the outside of your ankle bone and enters under your foot's arch from the opposite direction, sending out multiple strands of attachment as it runs diagonally towards your big toe. As the muscle fibres of peroneus longus cross over those of tibialis posterior they form a sling that acts like an elastic stirrup under your foot. If both arms of this cross-over stirrup are equally strong they help suspend the arch and also keep your ankle steady on the floor. It is a superb arrangement that points your foot in the right direction on the ground, so that the big and second toes—the prime movers of push-off—are best aligned for walking.

You will see later that the control of the inside arch is thwarted when your foot is not directed properly on the floor. Walking with

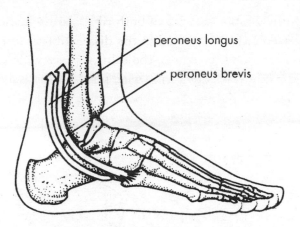

peroneus longus

peroneus brevis

FIGURE 9.4 Peroneus longus and peroneus brevis stabilise the outside of the ankle and help suspend the arch.

your hips turned out makes your feet roll over onto the inside border to get push off. This tends to press the inner arch flat and stretches both tibialis anterior and posterior. As the inner arch progressively flattens the talus also rolls inwards towards the floor.

The spring ligament also has a role to play in maintaining the foot's arch. This is a small, relatively insignificant but fantastically strong ligament on the underside of your foot. It spans the gulf between the calcaneum and navicular, running underneath the talus. It has a similar function to that of the tibialis posterior, but it works under different circumstances. The spring ligament holds the top of your foot's arch together and comes into its own when you land heavily on your foot, such as when you jump, run, hop or skip, when the compressive forces are so much greater and muscle tone alone cannot cope. Its tugging resilience prevents the arch splaying apart when your foot suffers explosive downward force. The muscles operate more continuously, exerting a low-grade tension to keep the calcaneum and navicular pinched into a crescent below the talus. The spring ligament spans the breach at the top of the arch and prevents the talus driving through to the floor. It too pulls the sides of the arch together, keeping the talus propped up as the pinnacle on top.

WHAT ARE THE ACCESSORY MOVEMENTS OF YOUR ANKLE?

As the keystone of your foot's arch, the talus performs the most subtle incremental action during weight bearing. In addition to the more obvious rolling out and back under the eave of the lower end of tibia, the talus undergoes a slight nodding–twisting movement as your foot takes weight. It moves inwards and downwards in a sort of screwing action, which is an ingenious way of dispersing load. It is the initial move, from the top of the arch down, that dissipates crushing loads through your foot. This small but vital component of accessory movement makes all the difference to your foot's ability to absorb shock.

As the instep flattens with bearing weight there is a slight rolling-in action over the inner border of your foot. Because the forefoot and toes are flat along the floor, the talus rolling in creates a relative twisting action between mid- and forefoot; only slight but there. During walking, the transient arch flattening also stretches the plantar structures that then spring back with elastic recoil as weight starts coming off. This elastic retraction provides another mechanism of forward propulsion, with the de-rotation of your foot contributing the almost imperceptible outward flick at push-off that adds an indefinable leaping lightness of step. Foot performance at its ultimate.

You can look down at your own foot as you walk and see the talus rolling in. As the foot takes weight, there is a momentary bulge along the inner border of the mid-foot, right at the top of the arch. At the same time, the calcaneum tilts slightly inwards as the weight comes over your foot. These small movements of the talus and calcaneum are but two of the accessory movements that help your foot absorb impact. But they are also the direction your foot goes when the inner arch collapses in.

Sub-talar movement is the other important accessory movement. Sub-talar movement allows you to absorb lateral instability on uneven ground. As your foot moves in and out laterally, the talus stays fixed in its mortice between your two anklebones and your foot moves under it. You can demonstrate this movement with your ankle up on your knee. Stabilising the talus with one hand over the front of your ankle, you can waggle the heel inwards and out with your other hand cupped around your heel. You will feel the dome of the talus wobbling slightly under the fingers of your right hand as you do so. All the lateral movement is happening at the sub-talar joint and you may notice there is more inward movement than outward. This leads to trouble.

HOW DOES THE ANKLE GO WRONG?

Both the congenital configuration of your foot's bones, including the way they stack around the arch, plus acquired muscle weakness can lead to trouble with ankles. Walking with excessively turned-out feet can also press your instep (or the inner arches) flat.

A turned-out foot strikes the ground with the outside border of your heel and then rolls diagonally forward, across the mid-foot to get push-off with the inside border of your big toe. Instead of propulsion being executed through the front pad of your big toe by the strong toe flexor muscles originating in the back of your calf, it is partly executed by peroneus longus and brevis, in an exaggerated sideways flicking action at your ankle. You saw in the previous chapter how the same turn-out causes problems with patella tracking. It also weakens the inner arch of your foot as tibialis anterior and posterior get progressively more attenuated. At the same time, their opposite number, the peronei muscles, get stronger and shorter. As your instep flattens, the talus screws in and down, similar to its transient action during the weight-bearing phase of walking—except this is for keeps. As weight leaves your foot, the talus does not spring back and the mid-foot does not de-rotate with a flick.

Over time, the front of the talus turns further and further in and down and your inner arch insidiously lengthens as it flattens. Neither muscles nor the spring ligament can hold the inside arch up and prevent your mid-foot from rolling in. The mechanical strain is great. Over time, all the structures of your underfoot become attenuated and weak and your foot hits the ground with a thud. At the same time, your foot becomes permanently twisted between the mid- and forefoot and your foot on the floor is as flat as a plate of meat.

Overaction of peroneus brevis with turn-out adds fuel to the fire. This muscle passes down around the outside of your anklebone to the base of the fifth metatarsal, about half way along the outside of your foot. In addition to lifting up the outside border, it suspends the much less significant lateral arch of your foot. When recruited by default to get push-off it becomes so strong it shortens your foot's lateral border and adds extra twist at the mid-foot as it flattens your instep. You will see at the end of this chapter that the 'foot twist' exercise reverses this condition by stretching the lateral border of your foot while at the same time re-establishing a better inner arch.

The anatomical design of your foot facilitates shock absorption and push-off but lays the groundwork for ankle injury. The foot dynamics predispose your ankle to turning itself under in the classical ankle-twisting strain. This is the most common ankle injury.

When your foot is at rest—off the ground and not bearing weight— it assumes a languid in-looking attitude with the soles of your feet seeming to face each other. Furthermore, your foot has greater inward range of movement than outward (as we saw above when waggling your ankle to demonstrate sub-talar movement). From the point of view of the bones themselves, there seems to be a bias towards your foot rolling inwards: the length of toes and metatarsals taper back from the front of your foot to the outer side, and the fibula is longer and situated further back than the tibia. All this makes it easier for your foot to roll on to its outer border and wrench your ankle.

These features of your foot have a singular purpose: to give the inner arch more gumption in its vital roles of stress distribution and push-off. In its natural state, your foot is almost pulled around into an inwards crescent that increases the power of the inner arch to resist flattening and also helps to make your big toe and, to a lesser degree, your second toe the chief orchestrators of push-off. All these points lead to trouble as far as accidental injury is concerned.

THE COMMON DISORDERS OF THE ANKLES

Sagging inner arches of the mid-foot

Sagging inner arches directly affect the function of your knees and the posture of your spine, though they themselves may not be painful. A fallen transverse arch, at the front of your foot, causes much more pain through excessive weight-bearing on the second metatarsal head (*see* the next chapter). Fallen medial arches look unsightly and cause cumulative wear on your skeleton by failing to dissipate impact and being poor at push-off. People with this problem galumph along with a heavy, flat-footed tread. Their gait is typically high-stepping as they compensate for poor propulsion by lifting their knees high. Poor arch support means that their feet slap the ground on heel strike and they roll in on their shoes, wearing down the inside heel rubber and stretching and distorting the leather of the back of the shoe. If you look at their unshod feet from behind, you will see their heels splayed out and their inner ankle-bones almost touching as they press inwards towards the floor. As the mid-foot twists inwards, the overactive peronei pull up an exaggerated arch in the outside border of their foot.

Impaired shock absorption of your feet transmits impact to your lumbar area, but more subtly, it affects the attitude or sit of your pelvis, which in turn discommodes your spine. In-rolling of your arches causes your pelvis to tip forwards, which may create an excessive scooped-hollow in your lower back and a slackening of your belly as your abdominal muscles switch off. Back disorders that are difficult to cure may be related to rolling-in arches and orthotics may be needed to speed rehabilitation. If fallen arches correspond to knock knees the orthotics may be wedged-up slightly on the inner border to help unravel your back problem from your feet upwards. The wedging also helps the tracking of the patellae.

Chronically twisting ankle

Although this is not a degenerative condition per se, an acute twisting strain of your ankle can become chronic if the original injury is bad enough. If the first injury is severe, your ankle rarely gets back to what it was. An accidental wrenching always occurs when the loaded foot buckles under at the sub-talar joint. Ongoing malfunction at the joint invariably leads to recurrent injury, and then to a worsening of the original condition. In its chronic state, poor ankle function affects all the other joints of your lower limb.

Take the first injury. The mechanics of this strain are this: the subtle inwards movement of your foot under the talus is forced to extremes by your body weight coming down hard on your foot in its twisted-under position. The immediate joint strain induced with its stretching of fibres and local painful swelling sets up a reaction where the surrounding muscles temporarily lock down the injured joint to take it out of action. The only trouble with this automatic joint-locking facility (known as protective muscle spasm) is that it can become overzealous, especially when fuelled by anxiety. For the sake of the future health of your joint, it is far better for swelling to be pumped away as soon as possible. If your ankle is not moved the swelling lies around in the tissues, stagnates and forms scar tissue. This explains why immobilising joint sprains for weeks in a cast is the worst thing you can do. Too often, the ankle finds itself caught in a web of scar tissue of its own making. Future movement is then tethered by these tight structures, particularly the lateral ligament of your ankle. This is how the plot thickens.

Your ankle cannot move freely during everyday movement, particularly the inversion (inward movement) that initially suffered the strain. Eventually, all inversion is lost and the slightest hint of your ankle turning under makes you collapse in pain. Even catching your foot on uneven paving can make you go down. Your ankle will swell again, with tenderness over the lateral ligament and wincing pain when you go to lift your foot off the floor.

Using crutches is not a good idea if your foot is left dangling limply. This will tend to make your toes drop, making it difficult to re-educate your foot to lift back. But more immediately, it will cause the swelling to collect in your foot, which will heighten the pain. Your toes may become puffy, even blue, despite the fact they were not injured. One option is to put your ankle in a cast for two to three days only, to control the swelling and to make it easier to get about. One thing is sure: if the original injury is not treated properly in the first instance, it will recur time and time again.

In its chronic state, the most striking feature is the thickness of your ankle. Whereas the other looks fine and delicately turned, this ankle is leathery and lacking its usual contours. All movements are restricted, including plantar- and dorsiflexion, though inversion at the sub-talar joint is obviously the most handicapped (twisting your forefoot around to see the undersole).

The ankle-twisting injury is more prone to recurrence than any other joint injury—with the possible exception of recurrent dislocation of the shoulder. It seems that once you've done it you keep doing it; your good ankle never attracts the same bad luck as the bad. As you know, it is the clenching-out of accessory movement and the resulting lack of passive acceptance of the jolts and bangs of everyday life that set it up for repeat injury: a walking accident waiting to happen. Only by restoring full accessory freedom can this joint be returned to normality.

WHAT CAN YOU DO ABOUT IT?

Again, like all joints the path to restoration follows the same signposts: restore universal joint freedom to the ankle complex and strengthen the muscle weakness, if there is any. Broadly speaking, lack of plantar- and dorsiflexion of your ankle influences your walking; it limits your length of stride and your efficiency of push off. On the other hand, paucity of lateral freedom at your ankle undermines your balance and the ability of your foot to maintain its arches.

Beginners

The arch raiser

This exercise targets the keystone of your foot's inside arch by pushing up the navicular bone from below. You will often feel an obstinate but pleasurably painful sensation in the soft part of your arch but, provided you have the mobility of your hips and knees to get into position, it is a fantastically effective self-mobilising technique, transforming your foot from a frozen hulk of bones into to a soft pliable arch. Your feet will tingle with gratitude when you get up and walk about, and you will be tempted to get straight down and do it again. The second part of the exercise mobilises the outer ankle and stretches the lateral ligament.

1 Sit on the floor and wedge your bottom hard into the corner with the wall.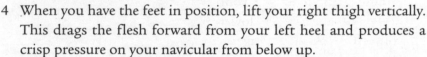

2 Bend your left knee and forcibly pull your left foot right into your groin, laying the top of this foot flat on the floor, as close in as possible.

3 Lift up your right foot and place it transversely across your left instep at the back of the arch, as close as possible to your left heel bone (you will need to tug in forcibly with your arms).

4 When you have the feet in position, lift your right thigh vertically. This drags the flesh forward from your left heel and produces a crisp pressure on your navicular from below up.

5 Wiggle your right knee left and right a few degrees, so the right heel presses into the left arch.

6 Continue oscillating the knee for 30 seconds then repeat twice.

7 Progress the exercise by keeping the right knee stationary and the foot trapped, and use your hands to lift the left knee off the floor, stretching the outer ankle.

Ankles-touching tiptoes

This exercise is harder than it looks. Its primary purpose is to balance the strength of the muscles controlling either sides of your ankles, in particular the elastic stirrup made by the crossover under your foot. When your arch is slung up equally from both sides it can better direct your foot straight along the floor, making it easier for your big and second toes to push off. The exercise also strengthens the muscles running the length of your underfoot, pinching the ends of the long arch together like catgut across a bow and raising it high. You should make a point of doing this exercise while cleaning your teeth. A minute or two a day makes a difference! You will notice it immediately walking down stairs, when your foot has the strength to lower your heel more slowly and lightly, so it doesn't thud.

1 Stand in front of a mantel-piece or hand-basin and hold on with your index finger—more to steady yourself than to take weight.
2 Keep your feet close together and your anklebones touching, then raise yourself high on your toes.
3 Hold this position for one minute without letting your heels fall apart then lower yourself back down again. Hard isn't it!
4 Repeat once.

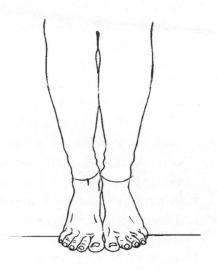

Intermediate

The foot squash

This exercise makes it easier to point your toe, which is often lacking after an ankle injury. Sitting on your heel with the top of the foot pressed flat forces talus out from under the eave of your tibia, like shelling a pea from its pod with pressure from behind. You can vary the mobilising forces by wriggling left and right on your heel, which prises the talus free and makes it easier to get out. If your ankle is very stiff, you will fudge it by turning the foot in, which you must resist. If your knee is too stiff to let you down onto your heel, use a cushion to get good contact; you need firm pressure on the heel. Sometimes the ankle feels sore and swells slightly after this exercise. This is no reason to stop, though you may rub an ice cube over your ankle to disperse swelling.

1 Kneel on your left knee with your toes pointing back. Your right leg should be out in front of you, its foot flat on the floor.

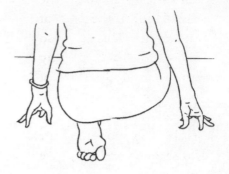

2 Balancing with your fingertips on the floor, lower your weight down onto the point of your left heel and sit on it. Make sure your foot does not roll inwards or outwards and keep your toes pointing straight back.

3 Sit like this for one minute then release.

4 Reverse the positions of your knees and heels and repeat with the other foot.

The Achilles stretch

This exercise may be unpleasant because Achilles tendons are extremely strong and slow to stretch out. You may feel your talus jamming at the front of your ankle, when it should roll back under your tibia. For this reason this exercise should follow the previous one; rolling the talus out further helps roll it back under better. The second part of the exercise, bending your knees forward, helps the tibia cover the talus. Yoga aficionados say this exercise stretches the veins of the lower leg and prevents varicose veins; you can certainly feel it either side of the ankle bones.

1 Stand on a stair facing up the stairs, if possible holding the banister. If you don't have stairs, find a step with at least a 10-centimetre drop. Stand right at the front edge of the step; literally hanging onto the edge of the tread with your toes.

2 Let your heels sink down to the next level. In your efforts to bring your heels down, don't let your bottom poke out.

3 Try to increase the stretch by pushing your knees forward to increase the angulation at the front of the ankles. This will also increase the pulling sensation at the back of your calves as you hang there.

4 Hold the position for 30 seconds and then rise up again.

5 Repeat twice.

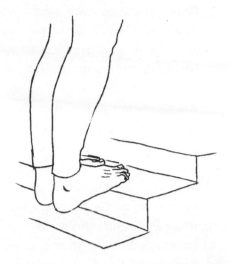

Advanced

The crossed-sole stretch

This exercise twists your feet inwards as far as possible and takes the lateral ligaments of your ankles to full stretch. When these ligaments are at full length it makes it easier to walk across uneven ground and provides lateral compliance when tipping sideways off uneven paving stones. It also stops your ankle muscles from seizing, which can bring you down in a heap. The uppermost foot receives the greater stretch in this pose, without the nursing protection of the other foot to dissipate the force. You will feel the tibial torsion in the knee. Make sure you have carpet or a soft towel under your feet to protect the bony prominences on the upper surfaces.

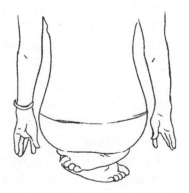

1 Kneel on the floor.

2 Turn your left foot inwards, laying the outside of your foot along the floor.

3   Place the top of your right forefoot into the saddle of the under-sole of your left foot, so that your feet are crossed.

4   Sit back on your feet so the weight of your bottom pushes your heels, particularly your right heel, outwards.

5   Hold this position for 1 minute then release by easing forwards and taking weight off your feet.

6   Reverse the position of your feet and repeat the sequence.

The foot twist

This exercise helps untwist your foot when overactivity of your peroneus brevis muscle has shortened the lateral border. This happens when you walk with your feet turned out and you roll diagonally inwards over your arch to push off with the inside of your big toe. The outward flicking action of your foot to propel you forward weakens the muscles of your inner arch and makes it even flatter. To make use of the new freedom gained with this exercise, you must learn to walk with your feet turned in—just a few degrees—to push off with the tip of your big toe. Make sure you have carpet or a soft towel under your feet to protect the bony prominences on the upper surface.

1   Kneel on your left knee with your right leg out in front of you, its foot flat on the floor.

2   Turn the toes of your left foot inwards and lay the outside of this foot along the floor behind you, with the ankle at a right angle.

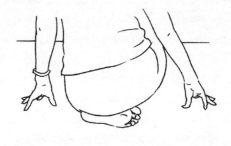

3   Lower your bottom down onto your left foot, especially on the inner heel section. Take some of your body weight through your arms. Depending on how much weight you let down, your ankle will be pushed into inversion.

4   Hold this position for 1 minute and then release by leaning forwards and easing off your foot.

5   Repeat once then change sides and repeat the sequence with the other foot.

Chapter ten
Your feet

WHAT IS YOUR FOOT?

The foot has five metatarsal bones that fan out from the front of the block of tarsal bones of your mid-foot. They spread forwards like a chicken's claw on the ground and connect up with your toes, which in turn continue beyond the sole of your foot.

There are three working arches of your foot that connect the three weight-bearing points: the heel, the base of the big toe and the base of the little toe. The medial arch was discussed in depth in the previous chapter. The lateral arch runs along the outside border and the transverse arch runs across the front of your foot between the first and fifth metatarsal head.

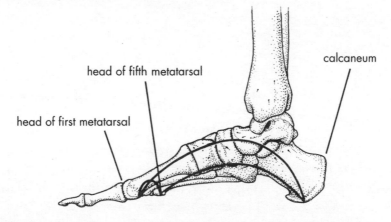

FIGURE 10.1 The three arches of the foot join the three major weight-bearing points.

The arches are everything to a foot; without them your foot would not be a foot. They help you with the very important roles of dispersing your body weight and propelling you forward with a spring in your step during the push-off phase of walking. Foot health is all about the vigour of your arches.

HOW DOES YOUR FOOT WORK?

Your foot largely works because of your toes, those funny little projections off the front. Humans don't use them as much these days; now we wrap them up and push them into shoes. But if your toes work well, your feet work well.

The most obvious job of your toes is to grab the ground and push you forwards and, let loose, they will do that very well. But they can do more. People without arms can manipulate objects with their feet almost as well as hands, which indicates how toes are blessed with far greater reserves of function than you ever call upon them to use. Indeed, they have exactly the same musculature as your hands and, though they have no opposing thumb, they are very effective if they have to be.

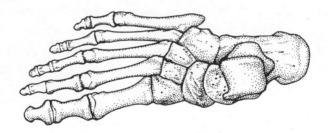

FIGURE 10.2 The foot spreads over the floor like a claw.

However potentially useful your feet might be, you usually only demand two jobs of them: weight distribution and locomotive push-off. Your toes contribute substantially to both of these functions because your toes and your foot's arches are intimately related. The muscles which work your toes, making them claw the floor to push you forward, also help bow your arches upwards and stop them flattening under load.

Broadly speaking, there are two sets of muscles that work your toes in grabbing the ground. First, there are the long flexors that come down from the back of the calf and span the underside of your foot to your toes. They curl your toes under, particularly the big toe, in a scrunching action. Secondly, there are the smaller, shorter toe flexors called the intrinsics. These originate under your foot and go through to your toes. They have a different action. They pull your toes to the floor and at the same time keep them straight; only bending the joint where your toe joins the foot, rather like the action of your fingers when playing the piano.

As you walk, you swing the non-weight-bearing leg through and strike the ground with your heel. Ideally, after heel-strike, your weight rolls straight forwards along your foot, over the mid-foot and on to the ball of your foot to your toes. At push-off, you claw the ground in a straight-toed action, mainly with the big toe and the second toe— correct ankle stabilisation having aligned your foot so you can do this.

A footprint in the sand reveals all there is to know about a foot. A perfectly balanced and dynamic foot leaves a finely etched scooped-out print but a severely dysfunctional foot will leave a great pad of a print, just like Yeti, the abominable snowman. The perfect foot leaves a delicately sculptured print, easily reflecting the three heaviest points of contact on the ground: a deeper impression under the heel; a less deep one under the base of the big toe, and a shallower one at the base of the little toe. Incidentally, you can always tell if the prints in the sand are that of a runner because the indentations at the toes will be deeper from the increased power of push-off.

WHAT ARE THE ACCESSORY MOVEMENTS OF YOUR FEET?

The important accessory freedom of your feet is the fine interplay between the small composite bones that make up the arch of your foot. The tension of the ligaments across the sole of your foot as well as the power of your muscles acting across the breach, offset the flattening effect of your body's weight bearing down on the top of the arch. With each step you take, the arch flattens slightly to absorb the shock. But as you start to push off, the arches are pinched together again by the muscles of your toes clawing the ground and by the elastic stirrup effect of your calf muscles working around your ankle. This means that during normal walking, the arch of your foot raises and lowers like the Sydney Harbour bridge, bowing up and flattening its famous arch. For this to happen there must be good mobility between all the bones of your foot, particularly the mid-foot.

Your bones must all be free to ride up and down independently of each other, rather like linked pontoons floating on a swell. Your bones must be free to open away from one another along the underside of the arch, forming V-shaped divots as the foot flattens. Internal mobility is also needed in a lateral spread across your foot so that the sole of your foot can mould itself to uneven surfaces on the ground in the same way that the palm of your hand can mould plasticine. The more mobile the foot the better. The more the individual bones can jostle and glide in relation to one another the more adaptable your foot will be. If accessory movement tightens up and your foot becomes semi-rigid, the dynamic arch qualities of your foot will suffer. As the arches collapse, a terrible saga can set in. The pain on walking, even standing, is an eternal lament.

Just as important is the effect this has on the rest of your body. If the arch is rigid, the shock-absorption qualities of your foot will be impaired. The ramifications from this travel far afield. If your feet slap the ground and there is no gentle letting down of your body, your entire skeletal frame will be shocked. The juddering will be felt right throughout your body and every joint will jump. Your skeleton and its joints will be prematurely aged.

HOW DOES A FOOT GO WRONG?

Binding your feet in socks and cramming them into shoes is one of the worst things you can do. This locks the toes away from usefulness and starts the steady decline. You should spend as much time as possible without shoes and socks, just so your toes can be free to participate and your arches can have a better chance of staying up. Toes entombed in leather are kept away from the warm earth. They cannot hook their farthest toe-pads around humps in the ground and your foot suffers. Imagine how useless your hands would be if they were encased in mittens all day.

Weakness of the intrinsic muscles of your feet immediately affects your toes and arches. With the straightening action of the intrinsics removed your toes start to claw. Unrestrained, the muscles that curl your toes under and those that lift your toes back make it impossible for your toes to remain straight. Instead of lying flat along the floor they scrunch up above the level of the rest of your foot. Walking bare-footed, they barely reach the ground. Your toes have completely lost their function of clawing and gripping the ground.

Often there are calluses on the top of your toes where the angled toe joints rub the inner surface of shoes. When a shoe pushes your toes down, they are forced to bear weight on their tips, even the nails, instead of the proper toe-pad on the undersurface. More importantly, the arches drop. This has all sorts of far-reaching side effects, not the least unsightly feet and at worst, crippling pain.

THE COMMON DISORDERS OF THE FEET

Flat feet

When the long arch on the inside of your foot falls, it is usually associated with a defect of ankle control with an in-rolling of your mid-foot. This was discussed in detail in the previous chapter. Here I will concentrate on the simplest manifestation of dysfunctional feet—the flattening of the arches.

Fallen arches are the scourge of the feet. Apart from looking bad, they can be almost unbearably painful with every step agony. As the arch presses down it causes a tired drawing and stinging pain along the under-side of your feet as the fascia and tendons of the foot are stretched.

The flattening of the transverse arch of your foot can be more painful. It is a different sort of pain and feels as if you are standing on a stone, right under the ball of your foot. The whole forefoot is in direct contact with the floor, in particular the front end (the head) of the second metatarsal.

Unlike the metatarsals for the big and little toe, the second metatarsal head is completely ill-equipped to bear weight. Most particularly, it doesn't have a fat pad underneath to cushion the contact of the bone with the ground and as a consequence it feels exactly as if you are walking on the bone itself. Over time, thick calluses of skin build up where the head rubs the ground, and this makes it even harder for this toe to work during walking. In extreme cases, the second toe remains cocked up and resting over on the others while the big toe deviates across and rests on the floor beneath it.

Feet problems for women can be much exacerbated by wearing high heels, especially if the shoes have a very narrow toe. Even if the foot works well enough unshod, it can be disabled by the shoe's cramped architecture, bunching the toes together and preventing them from pushing-off. The height of the heel also tips the body forwards and puts more weight on the front of the foot.

As a result there is an enforced lapse in the muscle control that suspends the transverse arch, just at the time it is needed most—when more weight than usual is coming down on to the ball of the foot. The transverse arch is flattened and a good proportion of your body weight is taken on the head of the second metatarsal. Even in the course of one shopping expedition or one cocktail party, it can feel as if your foot is on fire.

Bunions

This is the knob-like thickening at the base of the big toe. You may acquire this condition if you are born with an unusually short first metatarsal (the most medial long bone of the foot which connects with the big toe) and a slightly longer second metatarsal. Wearing bad shoes, especially high heels, can also cause bunions.

With the congenital condition, the longer second metatarsal head takes too much pressure during push-off. This hurts the bone and in time leads to progressive dysfunction of your foot. As your big toe gets weaker, the medial arch and transverse arches drop even faster. Painful calluses develop under the ball of your foot but more worrying is what happens to your big toe.

The big toe bends further and further in towards the other toes, at the same time making an unsightly bump along the inside border of your foot, where the toe makes an angle with the metatarsal. The big toe can also ride up over or go under the second toe. The cycle fuels as your big toe gets more helpless and the muscles controlling it get weaker. Like perishing catgut across the bow, the weak intrinsic muscles of the transverse arch allow it to drop and as a result the forefoot plays out across the floor.

Calluses—usually under the second metatarsal—are the hard and leathery layers of skin that build up in response to pressure. As the skin gets thicker your foot gets more uncomfortable, even though they are a protective response. Calluses need regular paring by a chiropodist but they will never go away until the function of your foot has been improved. In extreme cases, getting shoes to fit is a major problem because the large bump at the base of your big toe is almost impossible to accommodate. Flat sandals with an open-laced upper are the most comfortable but you often have to make your own arrangements by cutting holes in the leather.

It is awful to see someone with severe bunions trying to walk. They have a painful, hesitating totter, as they attempt to stay back on their heels, taking very small steps in a high-stepping action to obviate the need for push-off. Wads of cotton-wool and corn pads must be used to alleviate pressure areas inside the shoes in what can sometimes be a desperate situation. Neither shoes, chiropodists nor padding is the answer here. The solution, remote as the hope might be, is to get your toes and feet working again. With better understanding and better footwear, it is uncommon these days to see feet this bad.

But at the other end of the spectrum—for any normal mortal—better wellbeing can be had simply by having better feet. Reflexologists even claim that all the body organs have representations over different parts of the soles of the feet. They say that the workings of all our internal organs can be optimised by attention to the feet; that well-working feet make for a well-working system. It is certainly true that high-performance feet make an enormous difference.

WHAT CAN YOU DO ABOUT IT?

One of the first things you can do is take your shoes off more often. Your toes will rejoice at having all this freedom, and while initially they will remain scrunched up in the air, hardly getting any purchase on the ground, with each step, sooner than you would think, they will try to incorporate into a normal walking pattern. Uneven surfaces help; like soft squashy grass. And while you are walking make a deliberate effort to get your toes down, even to grab the floor, and *make* them propel you along. Wearing shoes without a back also helps because the toes have to work hard on the soles of the shoes to prevent them slipping off.

Beginners

Using the toes to lift the arches

This exercise encourages the straight-toed pawing action of your small intrinsic muscles, which at the same time lifts your metatarsal heads off the floor. This important action is usually invisible when swamped by the overall action of your toes pushing off but is a necessary integral part. It stops your toes scrunching up and keeps the toe-pads flat on the floor, while at the same time actively slinging up both your transverse and medial arches. Separating your toes and laying them down individually on the floor is an important first step; each toe learning to go it alone. Initially, it can be tediously frustrating because your toes feel so unresponsive, but it is worth working on, even though your feet feel as if they might cramp.

1 Stand upright with your feet parallel, about 10 centimetres apart.
2 Lift all your toes off the floor and separate them.
3 Lower them back onto the floor, spread as wide apart as possible.
4 Firmly plant your toes on the floor and lift the inside borders of your feet to

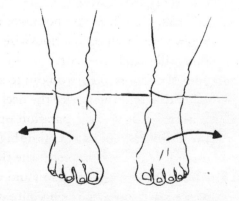

raise the inner arches, keeping your toes straight, not scrunched up.

5 Hold this position for 15 seconds and release.
6 Repeat six times.

The big-toe treatment

This exercise is most effective in the early days of bunion formation. It forcibly separates your big toe from the others and straightens the inward angulation at its metatarsal head. In separating the toe it also twists it through its shaft, which stretches the capsule, making it baggier. This makes correction of alignment easier. The second part of the exercises consists of using the muscles to actively work the big toe when you feel the tendons along the inside arch struggling to life. Small gains mean a lot in this exercise.

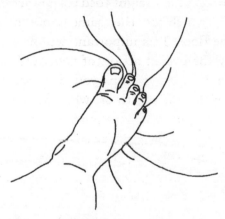

1 Using a yoga mat is ideal for this exercise because it creates drag. A towel is less ideal.
2 Lift your right heel and point your forefoot into the mat.
3 Screw your forefoot in a clockwise direction to splay the toes apart. This will runkle the mat.
4 Take the foot as far as you can to spread the big toe away from the other toes and then place the heel down on the floor.
5 With a small V-like separation opened up, try to press down on the under-pad at the end of the big toe to raise the forefoot and the underside of the bunion off the floor.
6 As the big toe loses traction and the gap closes, repeat the clockwise separation with the heel lifted up to six times, followed by the strengthening.

Intermediate

The dowling torture

This exercise is almost a bottled concentrate of sweet pain. Treading your feet incrementally forwards over a wooden pole mobilises the arches and gets into parts that nothing else can reach. It is not comfortable—you could say it is breathlessly painful—but your feet will feel amazing afterwards. You will need a long stick such as a broomstick, a walking stick or a piece of dowling 1.5 centimetres thick. It's worth buying the piece of wood especially for this exercise.

1 Stand in front of a mantel-piece or a table or any surface you can lean on to take your weight. Have the stick on the floor in front of you.
2 Taking some of your weight through your arms, hook your toes over the stick and then incrementally creep forwards, walking over the dowling.

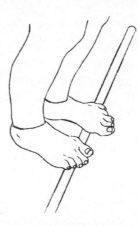

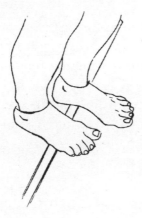

3 Take the smallest possible steps until you have passed right on over the dowling and stepped off the other side. Don't speed up when the dowling is under the painful parts of the foot.
4 Repeat twice.

Advanced
The toes push-back

This exercise means business. It pushes the toes back into full extension and makes you take weight on the tips of your metatarsal heads. It stretches the base of the capsules and prises the heads apart laterally, but its main value is breaking up the frozen plate-of-meat brittleness of your feet and getting your toes working individually again.

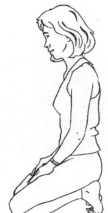

1 Kneel on the floor on your hands and knees.
2 Lean forwards on your hands and turn the tops of your toes under, with the toe-pads on the floor.
3 Sit back on your turned-under toes for 30 seconds.
4 Release and repeat the sequence twice more.

The toes push-under

This exercise stretches the upper part of your metatarsal head capsules, which shrink with a poor straight-toed action at push-off. If it is not dealt with, the capsular tightening contributes to your toes scrunching, so the knuckles perch above the rest of your feet. The leaning-back part of the exercise also stretches the long toe extensors, which originate in your shin and go through to the tops of your toes. You can feel these muscles being stretched across the front of your ankle as you lean back and tip your knees up.

1 Kneel on the floor and sit back on your feet, with the top surface of the feet flat on the floor under you.

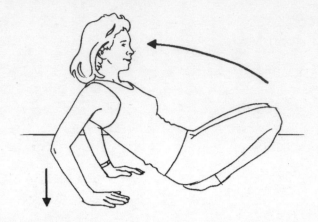

2 Place your hands on the floor beside you and, using them to push off, lift your knees as high as possible, pivoting on the front of your feet and toes.
3 Rock back as far as you can go and release.
4 Repeat four times.

The 30-minute daily regime

The right angle

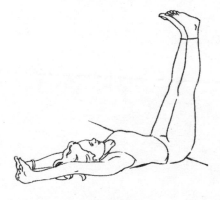

1 Find a clear space of wall with some uncluttered floor in front of it. Sit sideways into the wall with your bottom as close to it as possible.

2 Roll onto your back and swing your legs up the wall, stretching your arms out along the floor above your head. You should find yourself in a right-angled bend at the hips. Do not allow your knees to bend or your bottom to lift off the floor.

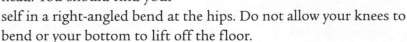

3 Hold this position for 2 to 5 minutes. You can make this exercise more taxing by interlacing your fingers and turning the palms away, above your head—keeping the arms parallel and not bending your elbows. You can also go one further by doing the 'angel's wings stretch' while in position by taking your arms down to your hips in a wide semi-circle, the backs of your hands in contact with the carpet all the way around. Try to breathe out as they go down and in as they come up.

4 To release, bend your legs on the wall, and round your back. With your knees bent, tip onto your side on the floor. Note that the longer you have been in this position, the more fixed you will feel on release. Make small wriggling movements on your side to soften your spine before getting up.

The floor twists

1 Lie on your back on a soft-carpeted floor with your arms out-stretched from the shoulders at right angles, palms facing down. Make sure you have a lot of space around you to do the exercise.
2 Bring both knees onto your chest, one at a time, and then take them over to your right so that they rest on the floor, keeping your knees high up to your body, as close to your chin as possible, and together. Your thighs should be parallel on the floor while you straighten your uppermost (left) leg at the knee.

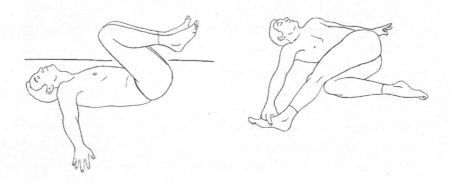

3 Attempt to hold the toes of your foot with your right hand. If you cannot reach the toes, hold behind your calf or knee, rather than bending the knee to reach your toes. Try to keep the palm of your left hand flat down on the carpet, which (often painfully) opens the front of this shoulder as the pectoral area stretches.
4 When in position, make small adjustments to get your upper back twisted back flatter, in closer contact with the floor.
5 Remain in position for 30 seconds, attempting to breathe into the bases of your lungs, then return to step 2.
6 Repeat to the other side and once again to each side.

The BackBlock

1 Lie on the floor on your back with your knees bent.
2 Lift your bottom off the floor by rolling up the spine, one cog at a time, until your body forms a straight line between shoulders, hips and knees.
3 Slide the BackBlock under your bottom and roll down the spine, coming gently to rest on the block on your way down. Make sure you don't position the BackBlock too high up your spine: it should *not* rest under the vertebrae themselves but under the sacrum, that hard flat bone at the bottom of the spine.

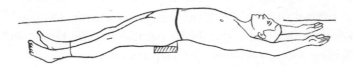

4 Gradually straighten each leg out along the floor by pushing your heel away from the block. Do not lift your legs as you straighten them as this strains the low back
5 Completely let go when you are in position over the BackBlock; the greater the relaxation the greater the segmental separation. Depending on your degree of kink, both at the front of your hips and at your low back, you will feel a pulling sensation in your low back, almost as though your legs are pulling the pelvis off the base of your spine. You should feel an agreeable discomfort, though it may sometimes be difficult to stay in position for more than a few seconds if the pulling is too great. It should not be agony but it should feel as though it means business; as if it goes straight to the nub of things.
6 After 60 seconds, or less if you cannot tolerate it, bend your knees slowly, one at a time, and lift up your bottom as you slide the Back-Block away. Lower your bottom to the floor, one cog at a time, just as you did when lifting up. It always hurts to raise your bottom off the BackBlock. Don't be fazed by this: the longer you have been lying there the more it will hurt to lift off.

7 Do the 'Knees rocking' exercise (below) for 30 seconds and 15 'Reverse curl-ups' (below) after coming off the BackBlock. If you fail to do these exercises afterwards you will be sore!

8 Repeat twice.

Knees rocking

1 Lie on your back on a folded towel on a carpeted floor.
2 Bring your right knee up to your chest and hold it with your right hand, then bring up the left knee and hold with your left hand.
3 Spread your knees as wide apart as is comfortable, still cupping them with your hands, and cross your ankles.
4 Oscillate your legs to your chest with your head relaxed on the floor. Do not tug at the knees causing the muscles of your neck to stand out. Feel your lower spinal interspaces opening at the back as your bottom gradually lifts further off the floor. You may alternate between rocking the knees up and down, then left to right and then in small circles, first clockwise then anti-clockwise
5 Continue for up to 5 minutes and repeat the exercise 2 hours later.

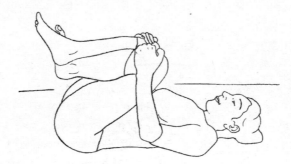

Reverse curl-ups

1 Lie on your back on the floor, pulling your thighs up to your chest with your ankles crossed and your knees apart. Interlace your fingers behind your head.
2 Without jerking, lift your bottom off the floor and your knees towards your chin and then return your thighs to the start position. Do not let your thighs go beyond vertical to the floor on the way down as this will strain your lower back.

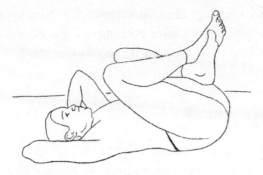

3   Repeat 15 times, bringing your legs up and down at the same speed, though you will find it much harder to lower the legs slowly. If you have a neck problem you will need to prevent strain travelling upwards by putting your hands, palms upwards, on your forehead instead of behind your neck.

The plough

1   You will need a pillow and a small stool or low chair. Position the stool about 45 centimetres away from the pillow on the floor.

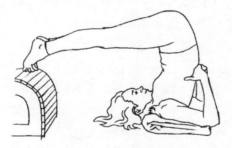

2   Lie on your back on the floor with the pillow positioned crossways under your shoulders and your head free on the floor. The pillow should be positioned to allow a step-down at the point where the thorax becomes the neck and this spares the neck from too much pushing under. The more uncomfortable the neck feels, the higher the pillow step-down should be.
3   Raise both legs up and swing them over your head so the feet rest on the stool behind your head. Make this movement smooth not jerky.

4 Support your bottom with your hands (arms bent at the elbow) and hold this position for as long as you can—up to 2 minutes if possible—relaxed and breathing evenly all the time.
5 Keep your chin tucked in and roll down your thoracic spine. Remove the blanket and then roll back and forth several times on your upper back to simulate spinal rolling.

The shoulder hang

1 Lie face down on the floor with a chair about 20 centimetres beyond your head.
2 Lift one arm at a time and place the flat of your hand on the seat of the chair. You may have to push the chair further away if you find the front edge is digging into your forearms.

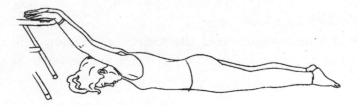

3 Straighten both arms at the elbows and drop your head through your shoulders to the floor. You will feel the pull diagonally up under your chest to the back of your armpits. Hang there for at least 60 seconds, longer if you can.
4 Slowly raise your head and lower your arms off the chair, one at a time. Rest for a while before repeating twice more.

The thoracic arms tangle

1 Sit towards the front of a kitchen chair with your feet on the floor and your spine held straight.
2 Take both arms out in front of you with the upper arms held parallel to the floor and both elbows bent at a right angle vertical to the floor.

3 Place your right arm over your left at the elbows so that the outer aspect of your arms touch each other.

4 Twine your forearms around each other so both palms are facing each other (albeit with the left palm lower down the forearm). Keep your upper arms held up parallel to the floor.

5 Now raise the whole tangled complex upwards, as high in front of your face as possible. You will feel a puffing sensation in your ribs where they attach to the spine in the upper back. The higher you go the more they will pull.

6 Hold for 15 seconds then relax.

7 Repeat 3 times then reverse the position of the arms and repeat another 4 times.

The up-and-down chair stretch

1 Standing in front of a chair, grasp the back of it for stability and place your right foot on the chair's seat.

2 Sink down onto your left knee on the floor. If the stretch is too great place a folded towel under your left knee.

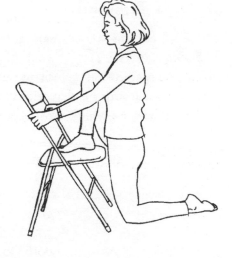

3 Keep your back straight and don't let your bottom poke out. If this is too difficult you may need to start with a lower chair or place a thicker mass under your knee (you could try a telephone directory).

4   Hold the position for 30 seconds and release.
5   Repeat with the other leg, then once more for each leg.

The sitting bowl

1   Kneel on the floor.
2   Press your big toes together, hook your thumbs around the inner side of your heels and pull those outwards.
3   With the heels widely separated and big toes together, lower your bottom down into the bowl-shaped hollow made by your feet.
4   Sit there for 1 minute with your bottom pressing your heels apart. During this time you can oscillate your bottom left and right to further force the heels apart.
5   Release and relax and repeat once more.

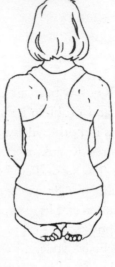

The toes push-back

1   Kneel on the floor on your hands and knees.
2   Lean forwards on your hands and turn the tops of your toes under, with the toe-pads on the floor.
3   Sit back on your turned-under toes for 30 seconds.
4   Release and repeat the sequence twice more.

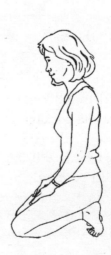

About the Author

Sarah Key has been involved with the management of skeletal disorders and problem backs for over three decades. She routinely sees patients in both Sydney (where she has a clinic in Bridge Street) and the United Kingdom, where she is the physiotherapist to the Royal Family. The second edition of this book takes its place beside *Back in Action* and *The Back Sufferers' Bible* and completes the trilogy in information and self-help for the skeleton's degenerative afflictions at its major points. In easy to understand layman's language, in a relaxed and inclusive style, all the mysteries of why joints become stiff and painful are laid bare. Sarah Key is married to lawyer Russell Keddie and has three adult children: Jemima, Harry and Scarlett.

Purchasing a BackBlock

To purchase a BackBlock, please send a cheque for £38 (price includes postage and packaging) to Blenheim Estate Office, Blenheim Palace, Woodstock, Oxfordshire, OX20 1PS, UK. Please make cheques payable to Sunsar Blocks Limited. BackBlocks come with instructions that must be strictly followed.

Instead of a BackBlock you can use a 5-centimetre stack of books. But the advantage of the Block is that its height can be varied easily. You start off with it on its low side (5 centimetres) and as you improve and it loses its bite you can progress to the next height (11 centimetres).

Index

Also available from Vermilion

Back Sufferers' Bible

By Sarah Key

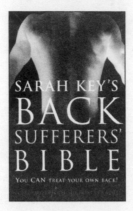

In accessible language, Sarah Key explains the cause of each spinal disorder and offers sound advice about how to treat the problem yourself. With easy-to-follow exercises and helpful advice on back pain management, the role of medication, the use of bed rest and how to return to work, this is essential reading for all sufferers of back pain.

£10.99   9780091814946